Foam Roller for Legs

A Step-by-Step Handbook to Stretch, Strengthen and Roll Out
Muscles, Eliminate Pain and Rehab and Rejuvenate Your Legs

DR. KARL KNOPF

Printed by: Createspace.com

10 9 8 7 6 5 4 3 2 1

Contributing writer: Rea Frey
Cover image: © Rapt Productions
Illustrations: pages 15–20 and 54–63 © TsuneoMP/shutterstock.com

July 2015
New York, New York USA

Please Note
This book has been written and published strictly for informational purposes, and in no way should be used as a substitute for actual instruction with quali-fied professionals. The author and publisher are providing you with information in this work so that you can have the knowledge and can choose, at your own risk, to act on that knowledge. The author and publisher also urge all readers to be aware of their health status and to consult health care professionals before beginning any fitness or health program.

table of contents

part 1

getting started

foam roller: the magic bullet?

Foam rollers were once used exclusively in physical therapy settings. In fact, Dr. Moshé Feldenkrais was credited with being the first person to use rollers for therapeutic purposes (e.g., improving body alignment, reducing muscle tightness, teaching body awareness) in the late 1950s.

Now they're used in yoga and Pilates classes to strengthen the body as well as relax and stretch tight muscles. They're also available in most gyms' stretching areas.

Some experts suggest that, if not addressed early, minor muscle imbalances (such as those tight, tender spots) can contribute to serious injuries or chronic dysfunction later on, which may require expensive therapy. Prevention is always easier and cheaper than treatment. Foam rollers are a wonderful way to address the above concerns while adding diversity and challenge to your standard exercise program.

Designing a balanced exercise routine that includes flexibility movements with strength training, cardiovascular exercise and relaxation can reduce chronic discomfort. Since foam rollers break up interwoven muscle fibers and help move oxygenated blood into those muscles, they're an excellent vehicle with which to release those tight spots in muscles (the technical term is "myofascial release") and return the muscles to a more optimal state. This can be done prior to exercising to improve range of motion, or after a workout to relax tight muscles and reduce soreness.

The beauty of the roller is that it's inexpensive and easy to use, and can be utilized to rehabilitate your body as well as prevent possible issues such as lower back pain and shin splints. *Foam Roller for Feet* provides you with numerous exercises to improve leg strengths and flexibility, as well as hone dynamic balance and mindful relaxation.

why use foam rollers?

The human body is designed in a remarkable manner and, if well maintained, will function efficiently for a very long time. Unfortunately, all too often we misuse or abuse our bodies, perhaps through activities of daily living or overuse. Whether you're highly active or sedentary, we all can benefit from a few minutes of light stretching and relaxation every day. A gentle, daily dose of movement keeps the joints lubricated and limber—motion is lotion.

More and more research in the field of exercise science shows that many of our chronic health issues can be positively influenced with corrective exercise. A former chief of orthopedics at Stanford University's School of Medicine once told me, "Modern medicine can do remarkable things, but we are nowhere close to rebuilding the human machine as well as the original equipment we were born with."

Today, therapists use progressive stretching programs and teach proper body mechanics as part of their standard arsenal to help ease clients' dysfunctions. Proper therapeutic exercise done regularly and performed prudently under the supervision of a trained therapist or personal trainer can be used to prevent injury, alleviate pain and restore your body to optimal levels.

You might already incorporate dumbbells, balance balls and resistance bands into your exercise program. Foam rollers are another tool that can provide an exciting and challenging dimension to your workout. One of the many great things about the foam roller is that it can be used by anyone, from severely disabled individuals to elite athletes. A simple adaptation can transform a basic exercise into an extreme challenge, thus allowing you to progressively ramp up the intensity of your routine and keep you from becoming bored.

A foam roller, used properly, is very effective for improving:

- Range of motion
- Core stability
- Balance
- Body awareness
- Flexibility
- Coordination
- Focus
- Body relaxation

The concept is that when you can perform an activity on a solid surface, you should progress to a less-stable platform in order to prompt your body to work harder. When you're on an unstable surface such as a foam roller, your body recruits more superficial and deep-lying muscles in order to maintain proper balance and body alignment. Some people often perform their normal exercise routine while standing or lying on a roller. By doing this, they not only isolate a particular muscle, they engage the whole kinetic chain, thus challenging all the major and deep-lying muscles.

Essentially, the exercises in this book, in concert with feedback from your health provider or massage therapist, can help you develop a better-balanced body. They'll keep your muscles toned and supple, which fosters improved functional fitness. They'll also demand that you practice proper posture and muscle alignment, which prevents joint dysfunctions and chronic pain. Joseph Pilates may have said it better: "Stretch what is tight and strengthen what is lax."

Lightweight and inexpensive, foam rollers can be stored almost anywhere, like under the bed or in a closet. Another advantage of foam roller exercises is that they can be done in the privacy of your home and you don't even need to put on exercise clothes. All you need is enough space to lie down and spread your arms.

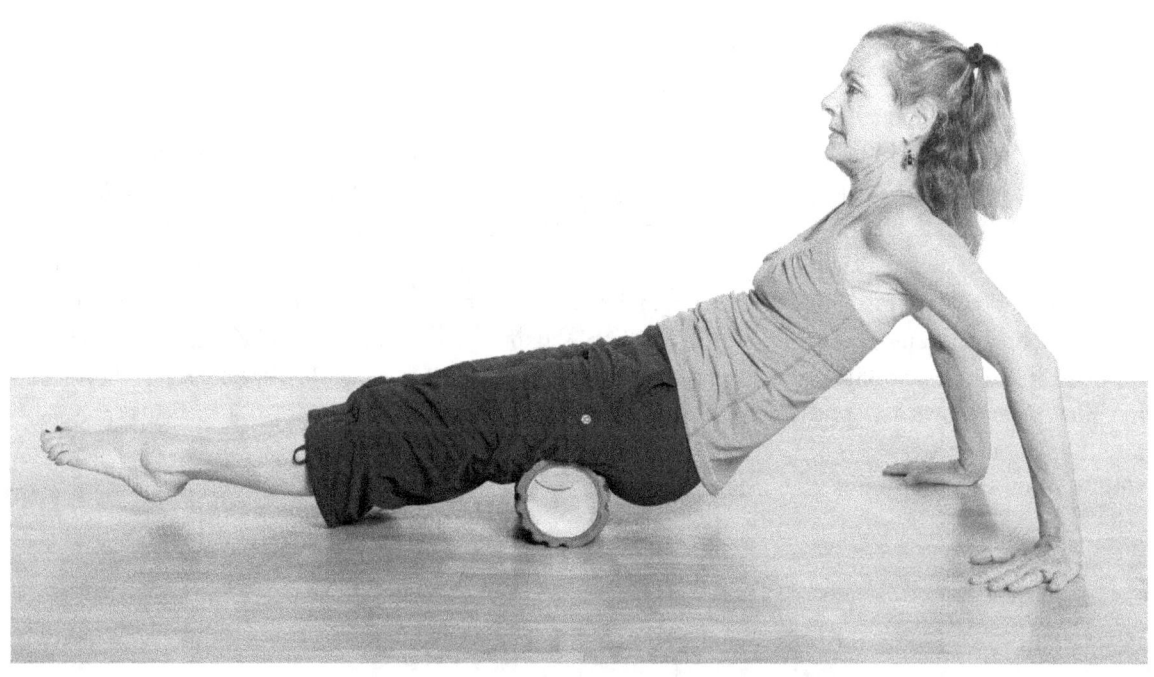

choosing a roller

Rollers come in a variety of shapes, sizes and densities and can be purchased online, at sporting goods stores and at physical therapy clinics. Selecting the type and length of roller you'll need is a personal decision, dependent on your height and weight, experience level and overall needs.

The most common roller configurations are semicircular or circular, either three feet or one foot long. Semicircular rollers, sometimes referred to as "half rollers," are flat on one side and curved on the other; they're typically three inches in diameter. Circular, or round, rollers are generally six inches in diameter.

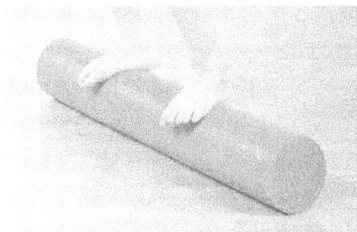

Circular rollers are more unstable (and thus more challenging) than their semi-circular counterparts. Note that you can place half rollers either flat side down or up. Having the flat side down is more stable than placing the round side down. Dense, firm rollers are good for self-massage, but if you're especially stiff, you may want to start with a softer roller so that your muscles can more easily acclimate to the pressure.

Circular roller.

The type of foam roller you're probably most familiar with is smooth. There are also foam rollers with small and large knobs on it to provide a deeper massage than a smooth roller can.

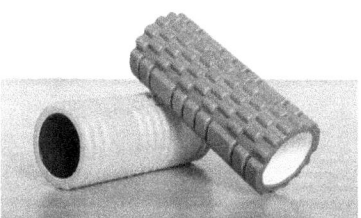

Foam rollers with small and large knobs for trigger point therapy.

Many exercises in this book utilize rollers that are three feet long, but some can be performed on shorter rollers. We refer to full-length half rollers as "FLHR" and full-length circular rollers as "FLCR."

If you're a beginner, a half roller is best. If you're looking to challenge yourself, you'll want a circular roller. Some people purchase one long roller and cut it to best meet their needs. Gyms often have various rollers you can experiment with.

Top: Half roller, flat side down.
Bottom: Half roller, flat side up.

before you begin

Using a roller looks like child's play, but utilizing it correctly is no easy feat. Before you roll your way to better posture, flexibility and relaxation, you should do all you can to make sure you're performing the exercises correctly and that your exercises and massages are comfortable and things you look forward to—they shouldn't cause pain. Always tune in to your body and stop if something feels wrong. Stepping, lying, kneeling or sitting on the roller should be your time to relax, refresh and renew yourself.

Safety
Foam rollers can be used by anyone, but if you've been diagnosed with a medical condition, it's highly recommended that you obtain personalized instruction from a trained therapist prior to engaging in a roller exercise program. It is ill-advised to use the roller if you suffer from the following: severe pain, poor range of motion/flexibility, poor balance, poor coordination, and/or the inability to get up and down from the floor unassisted.

It is always wise to ask your therapist to review this book and select the best exercises for you to start with. It's critical to train smart, not hard. Many of the conditions we suffer from took a long time to manifest themselves, so be patient in expecting results. Some chronic conditions such as arthritis can't be cured, but they can be managed very well with proper exercise.

Even if you're in good health, it's wise to have someone spot you when first getting started, especially when doing balance maneuvers. Also, make sure the area around you is free of obstacles. Be alert that if your muscles are tight and/or inflexible, the movements might be a little uncomfortable at first. Train—don't strain. It's better to do a little bit at first and progress slowly. Eventually, your range of motion will improve.

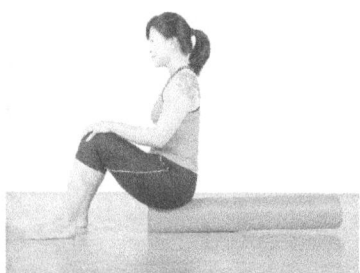
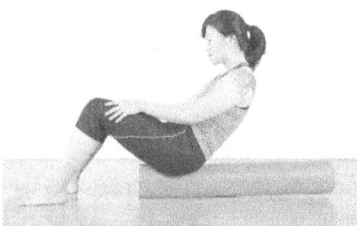
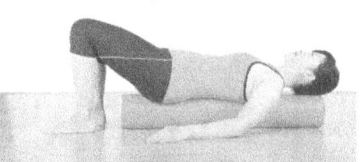

How to safely lie on a roller (supine).

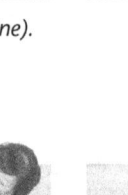
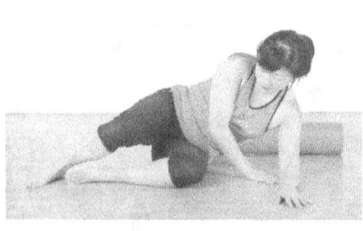
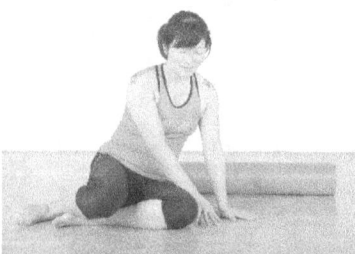

How to safely get off a roller.

When performing self-massage, only use the roller on muscle—avoid rolling on/over joints and bony areas. Additionally, massages should be done slowly. Enjoy the experience—don't create pain. In fact, "no pain, no gain" is insane!

Safety note: Always use the roller on a firm, non-slip surface.

Getting On and Off the Roller

There are a number of ways to situate yourself on a roller: lie face down, lie face up, sit, stand, kneel. Before you can do the exercises in this book properly, you'll need to know the right way to get on and off a roller.

Sitting

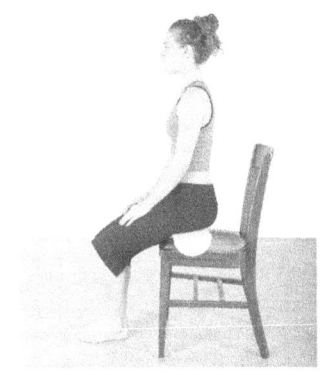

Proper sitting posture

Place the roller across a chair, sit on it with your "sitz bones" (the right and left tips of your pelvic bones, not your tailbone) and place your feet solidly on the floor. Your pelvis shouldn't tip forward or backward. Avoid overarching or slouching.

Lying

To lie face up on a roller (supine), start by sitting at the end of the roller. Keeping your knees bent and feet flat on the floor, slowly lie down, rolling your spine along the roller until the base of your skull rests at the other end. Use your hands as necessary for support. Maintain a normal arch in your lower back when performing all movements—do not allow your back to overarch.

To safely get off the roller, gently roll off the side of the roller onto the floor, turn onto your side, then press your hands into the floor to bring yourself to an upright position. If you're in good health and have a strong core, you can reverse the initial roll-down and come back up to sitting at the end of the roller.

To lie face up on a roller that's horizontal to you, sit on the floor in front of the roller and lie back on it, adjusting the roller to where it needs to be (hips, shoulders, etc.).

You can lie face down (prone) with the roller either horizontal or vertical to you. If the roller is vertical, straddle the roller in the manner of a push-up, then slowly lower your body onto the roller, aligning the roller from mid-pelvis to belly button to sternum. You can rest your head on the floor.

Kneeling

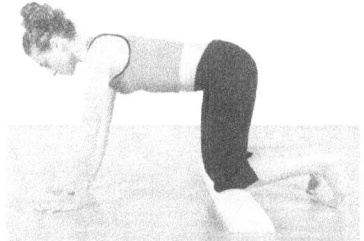

Proper kneeling position.

Place your knees on the roller and your hands on the floor so that you're on all fours. When the exercise asks you to put your hands on the roller, just reverse the process. If the exercise asks you to kneel upright, you may want to do this next to a chair or wall for support. Keep the area clear of objects for when you lose your balance.

Standing

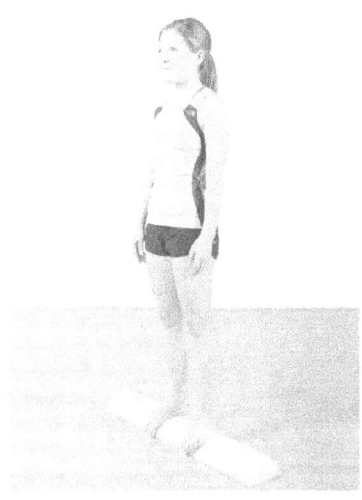

Proper standing posture.

When standing on the roller, never compromise good posture to gain balance. Always maintain a neutral spine:

From a side view, your ears are stacked above your shoulders and your shoulders are aligned with your ankle bones.

- Keep equal weight on both feet and over the ball of your foot and heel.
- Your knees are slightly bent.
- Your pelvis should be in neutral position, neither tilted backward or forward.
- The span from your belly button to breastbone is long and lean.
- Gently pull back your shoulder blades.
- Your chin is a fist distance from your chest.

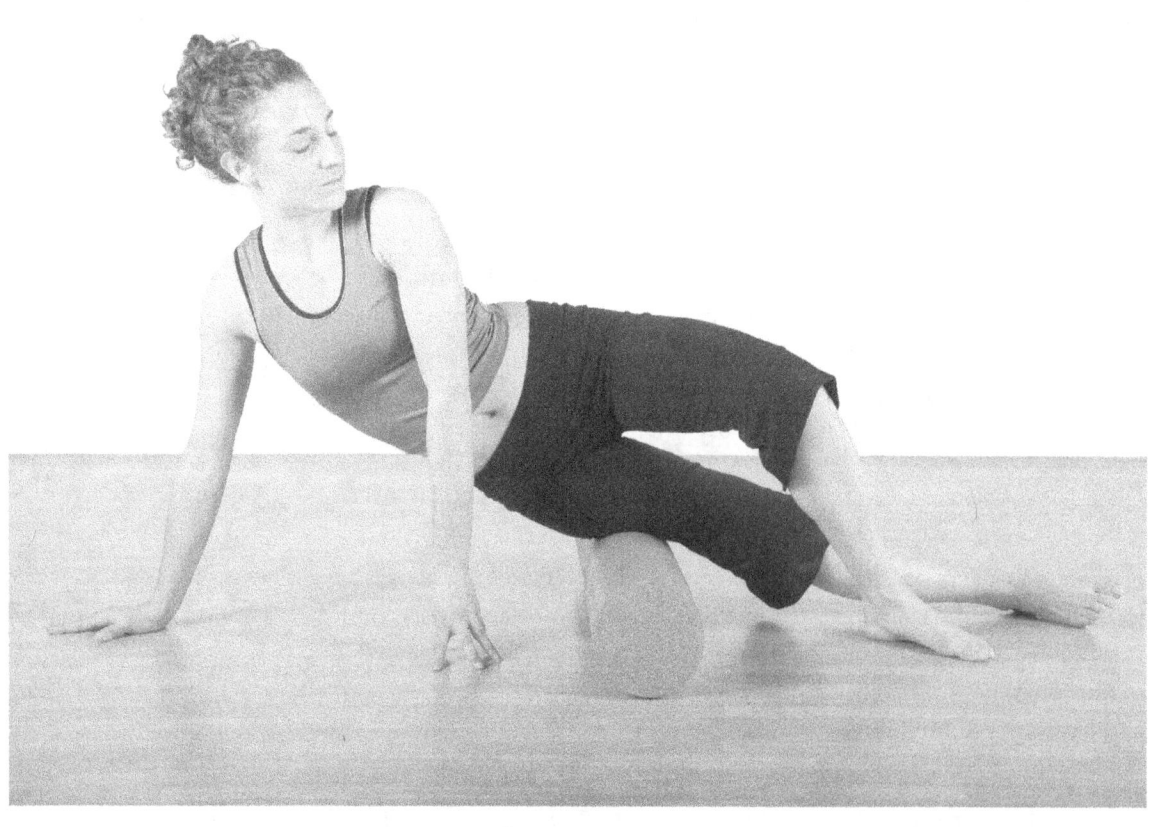

how to use this book

This section of the *Foam Roller for Legs* presents two programs for leg strength and flexibility. You may notice that there is the omission of repetitions (reps) and sets. Unfortunately, most of us are still dialed into the outdated mindset of "How many do you want me to do, Coach?" When deciding how many reps or sets of these foam roller exercises to do, the key is to forget about the number of reps you need to do and, instead, focus on maintaining proper posture and engaging the targeted muscles. You'll get better results by tuning in to your body and performing the movements with correct biomechanical form.

If that concept is too far out for you, start with 3–5 reps for active movements or 10 seconds for static positions. As the movement become easy, add more reps or think of other methods to challenge yourself. Aim to increase the number of reps to 30 or hold static poses for 30–60 seconds. Remember, more is not necessarily better. Also, when performing the movements, focus on breathing and being centered.

The exercise instructions will call for full-length half roller (FLHR), full-length circular roller (FLCR) or half-length knobbed circular rollers. Generally, we'll start with the least challenging option (typically a FLHR with the flat side down); incorporating the FLCR is oftentimes the most challenging. However, feel free to use the one you have on hand or that's appropriate for your ability level. The FLHR is easier to control and maintain your form and balance on, but most gyms only have FLCR rollers. Be aware that it's very easy to lose proper alignment on a FLCR if you're not careful.

The Exercises

This book features foam roller exercises from a variety of positions: seated, lying, kneeling and standing. Since one of the original uses for the roller was to provide a self-administered, deep-tissue pressure massage, often called "myofascial release," we also include a few using the smooth and knobbed rollers.

The entry-level seated exercises are performed while sitting in a chair. They're designed to familiarize you with the roller and to foster improved posture and core stability.

In physical therapy or at the gym, you'll most commonly use the foam roller while lying on your back (or supine position). We also present a few exercises in which you're face down (prone). These exercises may look simple, but they're amazingly challenging. If you're at all self-conscious, find a private space to learn them. It'll take time to be able to maintain proper alignment and stability on the roller. Think PP = perfect posture. Perfect form is more important than speed or number of reps. For exercises on your back, you may want to start with a half roller, flat side down. As you become more comfortable, flip the roller over and try the exercise from the less stable position. Once you're proficient at that stage, try a full circular roller, and once you're proficient at that, rest your feet on a pillow or any unstable surface to challenge yourself even more.

The for standing exercises, all done while standing on a foam roller, are difficult and challenging. You'll want to start with a half roller flat side down. This standing exercises are best suited for people in great physical condition who also have excellent balance. Some of the movements will be done on a full-length circular roller. Since all the standing exercises necessitate a requisite level of balance, you might want to place a chair alongside you, stand in a doorframe or have someone spot you to provide support. The main focus of these standing exercises is to improve static and dynamic balance as well as core stability.

Initially, it's useful to perform the movements in front of a mirror so that you can watch yourself, or ask a friend to observe you and kindly make corrections. If you do these moves with someone, remember that every body is unique—a movement that's easy for your flexible friend may be impossible for you.

With self-massage and release exercises in this book, you determine the amount of pressure you receive. However, if you've had a recent injury, consult your health care professional prior to performing any self-massages or releases. Here are some things to consider with regards to self-massageand releases.

- A firm, circular roller (knobbed or smooth) is best.
- Apply pressure only to soft body tissue, not bony areas such as joints.
- Start at the area closest to the body and roll out away from there.
- Maintain perfect posture at all times.
- Be alert to the difference between pain and discomfort.
- Don't cause pain or perform a prolonged massage on a tender area—be gentle.

introduction to leg muscles

On average, our legs constitute nearly 45 percent of our total height. That's right, almost half the human body is made up of legs. If you are an athlete that utilizes your legs for your sport of choice, whether that's something low impact on the scale like yoga or swimming or high-impact like running or soccer, you're probably keenly aware of how much power you ask your legs to produce. What's more, you're probably also aware of just how strong yet sensitive your leg muscles are. Cramps, soreness and even muscle pulls are the name of the game for leg-intensive athletes. So let's take a couple of minutes to get familiar with all the various muscles that make up the lower body.

Glutes

The buttocks consist of the *gluteus medius* and the *gluteus maximus*. The majority of the glutes stem from the *gluteus maximus*, which extends the hip joint and moves the leg backward.

Gluteus Maximus

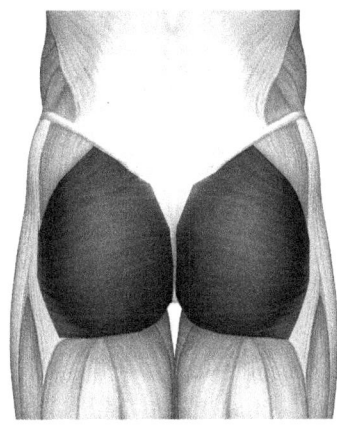

The strongest muscle in the body, the *gluteus maximus* connects the sacrum, ilium, and coccyx to the femur and assists in extending the thigh. When a person walks, runs, or climbs, the *gluteus maximus* helps the leg straighten at the hip and helps a person stand from a seated position. In addition, the *gluteus maximus* helps someone hold isometric positions, such as squatting, for long periods of time. The glutes can handle a lot of force and should be thoroughly strengthened to build and protect the lower back, core, and hips.

Gluteus Medius

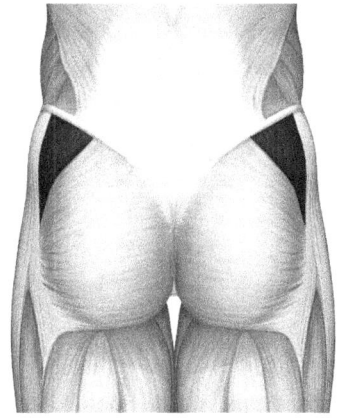

Located underneath the *gluteus maximus*, the *gluteus medius* abducts and stabilizes the hips through activities like walking. The *gluteus medius* helps move the thigh out to the side and, just as its name suggests, rotates the thigh medially. The *gluteus medius* can be strengthened by abducting the hip and working smaller, less intense movements than the *gluteus maximus*, such as leg raises and glute kickbacks.

Strong glutes are responsible for moving the hips, squatting, lunging, jumping, running, and being able to hold isometric positions. Most lower-body or full-body sports and activities require using the glutes. Since the glutes are the strongest muscle in the body, well-defined glutes are tantamount to healthy hips and lower back.

Glutes and hips need to be stretched to prevent lower back tightness. Often, when someone complains of lower back pain, it can directly be correlated to tight glutes or hamstrings. Balancing, strengthening, and stretching the glutes and hips should be worked into a regular routine. Warming glutes up with easy air squats, hip mobility exercises, such as a swimmer's kick, light walking or jogging can help prepare for more intense movements. Stretching glutes at the end of a workout via yoga movements, rolling on foam rollers, or through static stretches is necessary for muscle and joint health.

Glute tears are rare. Because the muscle is so large, it's important to focus on other movements besides squats and lunges to hit the smaller muscles, such as the piriformis and the gluteus minimus. While squats, step-ups, and lunges are popular glute moves, hip bridges, glute extensions, kickbacks, and other bodyweight movements can help shape and tone the backside, leading to a more symmetrical physique.

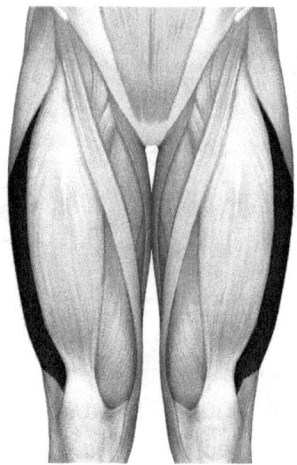

FOAM ROLLER EXERCISES
Gluteal Massage, page 46
One-Leg Balance, page 43

Thighs

The thighs consist primarily of the four-headed quadriceps femoris. Three of its heads, the *rectus femoris*, *vastus lateralis*, and *vastus medialis*, are responsible for extending the knee and flexing the hip.

Rectus Femoris and Vastus Medialis

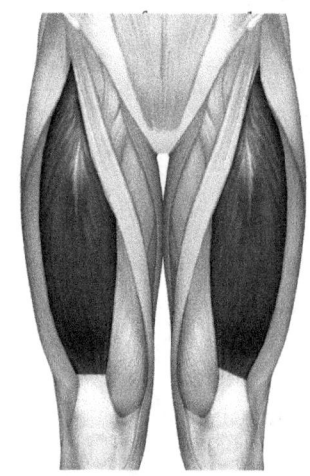

Rectus femoris

The *rectus femoris*, which is located along the front of the thigh and inserts at the patella (knee cap) via the quadriceps tendon, is connected to the hip and helps extend the knee. The *rectus femoris* helps contract the thigh and can actually flex the hip.

Vastus lateralis

The *vastus lateralis*, which is located on the side of the thigh, composes the majority of the quadriceps and extends the knee. The quadriceps' tendon attaches directly to the patella, which helps protect the tendon from wear and tear, allowing for normal knee range of motion. The *vastus medialis* extends the length of the thigh and runs medially toward the inner thigh. The *vastus medialis* extends the knee, adducts the thigh, extends and externally rotates the thigh, and stabilizes the patella.

These muscles work together and form the large sweep of the thigh. The quads can be strengthened in a variety of ways, such as running, jumping, squatting, lunging, climbing, and so on. Stretching and rolling the quads and keeping the hamstrings equally strengthened can prevent knee injuries and quadriceps tears. Groin pulls, or tears in the adductor tendons, however, can be quite common. Making sure to thoroughly warm up, work accessory muscles, and cool down properly is all part of keeping the thighs healthy.

Pectineus

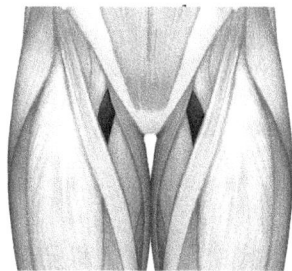

The *pectineus*, which attaches from the pubic bone to the femur, flexes and adducts the hip toward the center of the body and assists with hip flexion. The *pectineus* can be strengthened with movements such as lateral lunges, side lying hip adduction, hip adduction, and lying hip flexion.

Tensor Fascia Latae

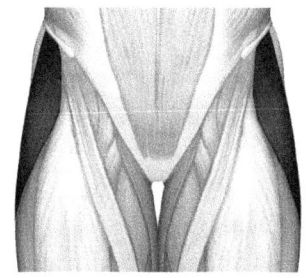

The *tensor fascia latae* is a tiny muscle that helps steady the thigh when standing upright. It is used primarily in activities such as skiing and horseback riding. Issues with the pelvis may arise if this muscle becomes strained or shortened.

Sartorius

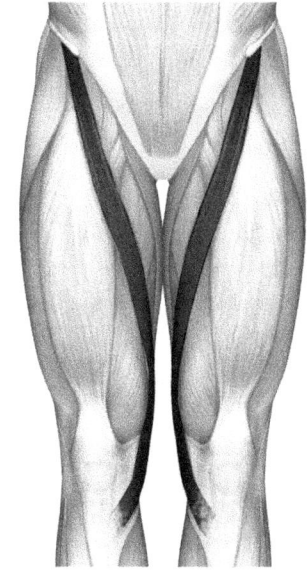

The sartorius is the longest muscle in the human body. It stretches the entire distance of the thigh and flexes, adducts, and laterally rotates the hip while flexing the knee. The sartorius also helps drive the ankle and foot toward the knee of the opposing leg. This muscle allows movements such as crossing your legs or looking at the sole of your foot.

Adductor Longus

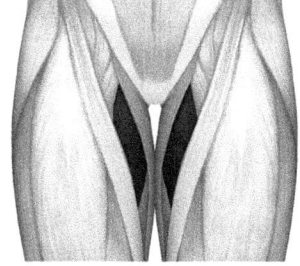

The *adductor longus* attaches from the pubis to the femur and appears as a long, triangular muscle. It helps flex, rotate, and move the thigh inward for a variety of movements.

Gracilis

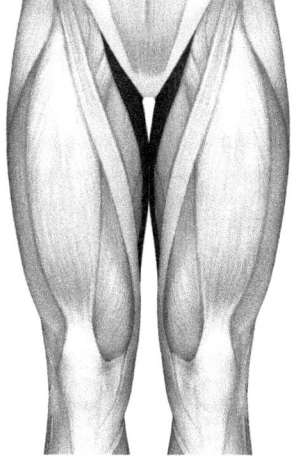

The *gracilis* attaches from the pubis to the tibia and adducts the thigh. It also medially rotates and flexes the leg at the knee.

All of these muscles work together to protect the knee and help with everyday movements as well as athletic endeavors. While you can isolate certain muscles in the thighs, such as the inner and outer thighs and the quadriceps, they all work together to complete compound movements. Making sure to adequately warm up the thighs through dynamic movements is an important part of training the legs, whether through strength training or conditioning. Static stretching can be performed after exercise, paying special attention to the hips, glutes, hamstrings, quads, and inner thighs. Strains, sprains, and tears can occur in the thighs if not properly warmed up. There are a variety of exercises that can be performed for strengthening the thighs, such as most sports, running, strength training, dancing, and even everyday activities like walking or climbing stairs.

FOAM ROLLER EXERCISES

Quad Stretch, page 48

Standing Mini Squat, page 39

Quad Massage, page 47

Inner Thigh Massage, page 50

Hamstrings

The hamstrings run the length of the back of the leg from the pelvis to the tibia and fibula. They act as the main flexors of the knee. The three main muscle groups of the hamstrings are the *semimembranosus*, *semitendinosus*, and the *biceps femoris*, which is considered the "two-headed muscle" of the hamstrings.

Semimembranosus

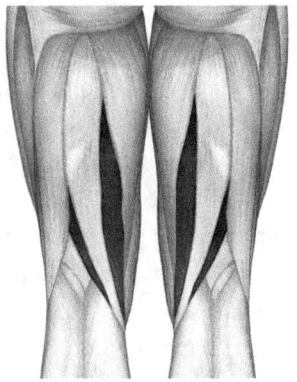

The *semimembranosus* is the innermost muscle in the back of the thigh. It flexes and rotates the leg medially, as well as extends the thigh. The *semimembranosus* is actively engaged whenever the leg curls in toward the body or the hips extend.

Semitendinosus and Biceps Femoris

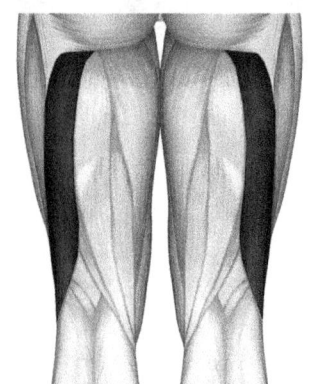

Biceps femoris

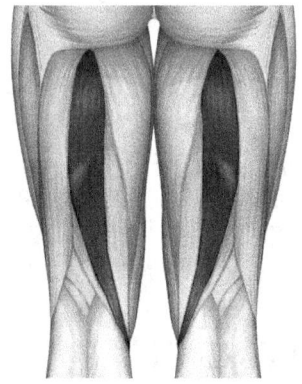

Semitendinosus

The *semitendinosus* appears as a bandlike muscle in the hamstrings and acts as a strong tendon, flexing and rotating the leg to extend the thigh. The *biceps femoris* has both a short head and a long head. Both heads attach to the pelvis and the thigh bone and connect on the lateral side of the back of the thigh. The long head flexes and rotates the leg laterally. It also extends the thigh. All three of these muscles work together to perform normal hamstring functions, such as curling the leg toward the glute and extending the hips up.

Iliotibial Band

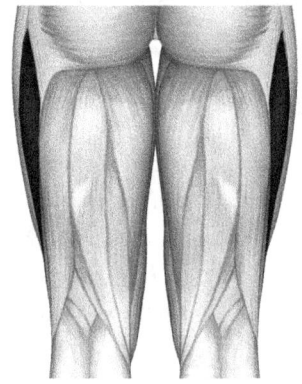

The iliotibial band, or IT band, and *adductor magnus* are also parts of the hamstrings. The iliotibial band, also known as the iliotibial tract, connects numerous muscles in the thigh. It abducts, medially rotates, and flexes the thigh. It also helps support the extension of the knee when biking, walking, running, and even standing. The connective tissue contains collagen, which allows the iliotibial band to be incredibly strong in some directions and weaker in others. Many people experience ITBS, or iliotibial band syndrome, which stems from friction and causes inflammation, irritation, and pain. Resting, icing, rolling, massage, and even compressing the IT band can make a tremendous difference for pain-free activities. Endurance runners often experience issues with the iliotibial band.

Adductor Magnus

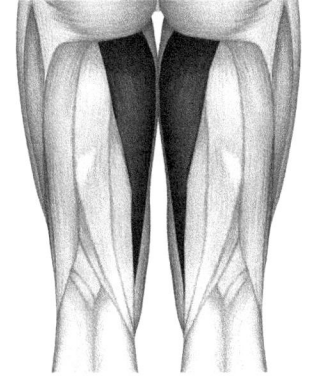

The largest of the three adductor muscles, the *adductor magnus* inserts at the femur and runs up to the pelvic bone. The *adductor magnus* medially rotates the leg and adducts the hip.

Working the backs of the legs and the glutes can strengthen all the muscles that comprise the hamstrings and is vital for a stable knee joint. Strong, well-balanced hamstrings can reduce the likelihood of injuries to ligaments during sports or recreational activities. Properly warming up the hamstrings with dynamic stretches and static stretches post-workout, as well as working the hamstrings as much, if not more, than the quadriceps, will result in

a more symmetrical appearance and less chance of a knee injury.

Hamstring tears are common and can be avoided by comprehensive strength training and working toward proper activity level by refraining from performing explosive movements before the body is ready. Any movement that involves kicking or curling the leg behind the body, thrusting the hips in an upward motion, or bending over from the hips requires significant use of the hamstrings.

FOAM ROLLER EXERCISES

Hamstring Release (chair), page 28

Hamstring Massage, page 52

Iliotibial Band Massage, page 49

Calves

The calves are the bulky muscles at the lower posterior part of the leg, above the ankles and feet. The calves contain numerous muscles that work together to allow movement of the ankles and feet.

Gastrocnemius and Soleus

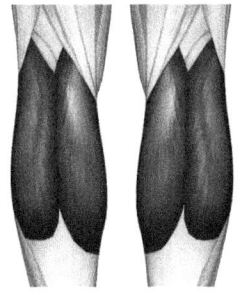

The gastrocnemius muscle

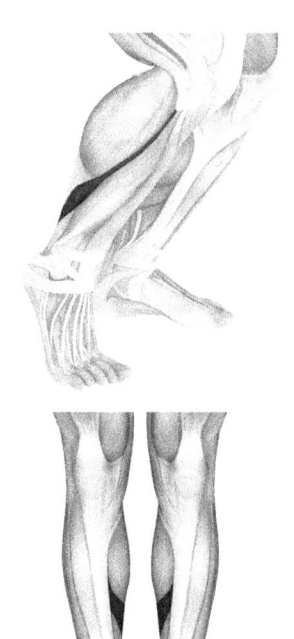

Two views of the soleus muscle

The *gastrocnemius* and *soleus* form the Achilles tendon and allow the ball of the foot to push down and off from the ground. The *gastrocnemius* consists of the lateral and medial heads. When running or walking, the *gastrocnemius* helps push the body forward, flexes the leg at the knee and is a plantar flexor as well. This is the main muscle people focus on when strengthening or stretching the calf.

Tibialis Anterior

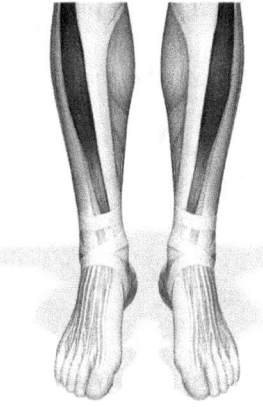

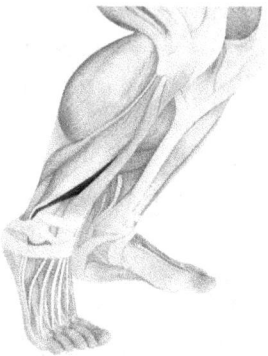

Peroneus brevis

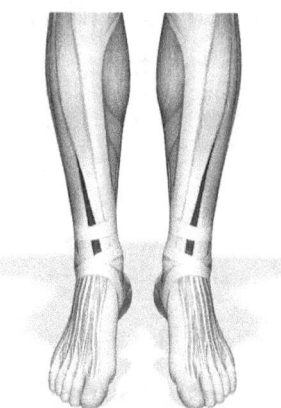

Flexor hallucis longus

The calf also includes the *tibialis anterior*, which allows dorsiflexion of the foot and helps stabilize the foot, especially when walking. The dorsiflexion of the *tibialis anterior* allows the toes to pull off the ground and moves the foot toward the body's midline. The *tibialis anterior* also helps when balancing on one foot and comes in handy when doing yoga, ballet, or activities that require exceptional balance.

Peroneus Longus and Peroneus Brevis

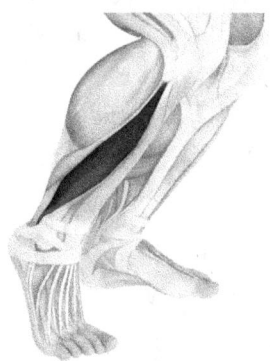

The peroneus longus

The *peroneus longus* is a major muscle of the calf and plantar flexes and turns the foot outward at the ankle. The *peroneus longus* helps the *gastrocnemius* and *soleus* to point the toes, stand on one foot, shift weight over the planted foot, and keep the toes in the correct position for any given movement. The *peroneus brevis* extends and abducts the foot, which is important for foot rotation in sports like boxing and dancing.

Extensor Digitorum and Flexor Halluces Longus

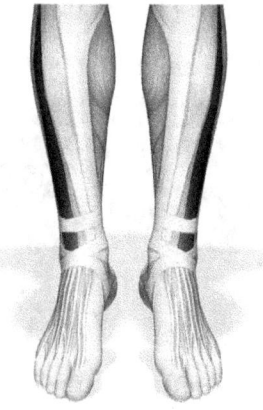

The extensor digitorum

Located behind the *tibialis anterior* at the outside of the lower leg, the *extensor digitorum longus* provides dorsiflexion of the foot, eversion of the foot, and full extension of the toes. The *flexor hallucis longus* are muscles used for extending the big toe, which aids in balance and pivoting on the feet.

Together, all of these muscles form the calf, which is responsible for movements of the ankles and toes. Calves allow elevation of the toes, pivoting, rotation, and extension. The calves are mandatory in activities like walking, running, reaching for something, squatting, and balancing.

Calves can easily be strengthened with bodyweight by elevating onto the toes and outwardly or inwardly rotating the feet. Weight can be added for toe raises as well for those who wish to add size to the calf muscles. Jumping rope, running, sprinting, or bouncing on the balls of the feet are wonderful conditioning and strength exercises for the calves.

In order to prevent an injury, calves should always be stretched and warmed up before ballistic movements. Calf pulls or tears are common and can be avoided with regular strength training and proper stretching post-workout. Making sure to move the feet and calves, especially when on long plane rides, to avoid clots and cramping is mandatory. Ingesting plenty of potassium to avoid muscle cramps—which commonly occur in the calves— also helps keep the calves healthy.

hamstring flexibility program

According to some experts, the inability to touch the toes can contribute to lower back pain. Whether you're active or sedentary, you probably have tight hamstrings. This routine offers some simple methods to improve flexibility in the backs of your legs.

HAMSTRING FLEXIBILITY PROGRAM

PAGE	EXERCISE
46	Gluteal Massage
51	Total Calf Release
52	Hamstring Massage
33	Plank to Pike
47	Quad Massage
35	Pointer Sequence
49	Iliotibial Band Massage
50	Inner Thigh Massage

balance and lower-limb flexibility program

This routine addresses balance, leg strength and lower-limb flexibility.

SKIING PROGRAM

	PAGE	EXERCISE
	38	Standing Slide
	39	Standing Mini Squat
	40	Standing Ball Pick-Up
	41	Tightrope Walk
	43	One-Leg Balance
	42	Rock and Roll
	45	Compound Skiing
	44	Skiing
	52	Hamstring Massage
	33	Side Salutation
	46	Gluteal Massage
	51	Total Calf Release

part 2

exercises

Goal: To improve neutral spine awareness and foster ankle flexibility

STARTING POSITION: Sit upright in a chair. Place a FLCR on the floor and rest your feet on top.

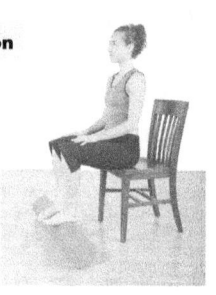

1–2 Slowly and gently roll your ankles forward and back. Remember to stay in your pain-free zone.

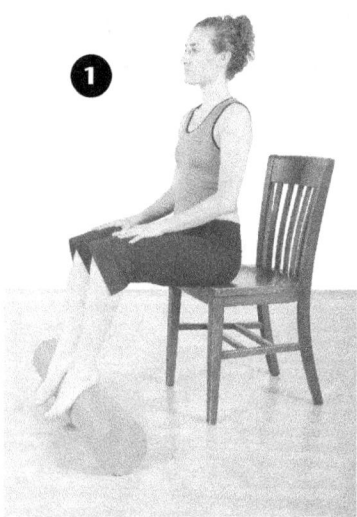

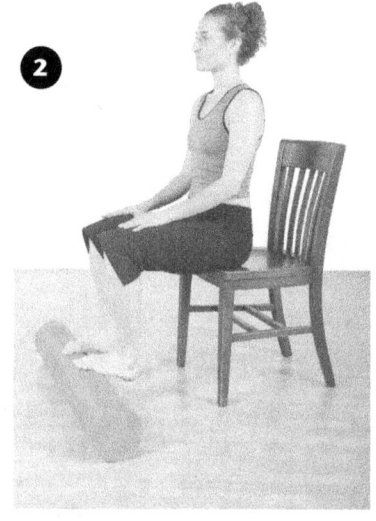

This can be performed using one foot or both feet at a time. Make sure you do this movement in a sturdy chair.

STARTING POSITION: While seated, place the knobbed roller under one foot.

starting position

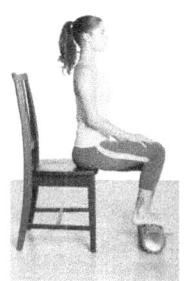

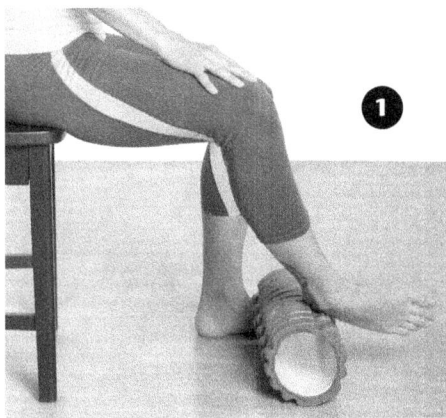

1-2 Apply pressure, rolling and pressing the bottom and sides of your foot over the roller, stopping at tight areas and holding for a few moments. Use your intuition to know how hard to press and how long to hold. Aim to hold the position for 5 to 30 seconds. Relax and repeat as desired. Breathe slowly and fully.

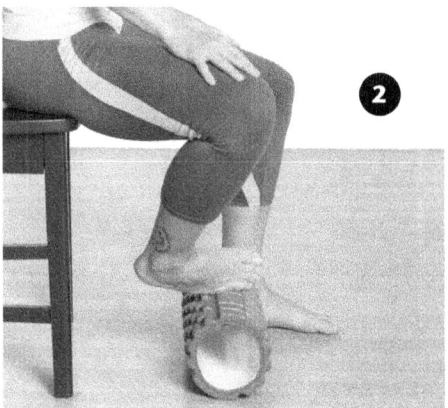

This can be done with one or both legs at the same time.

THE POSITION: Sit in a chair and place the knobbed roller under one thigh. Gently roll and press your leg along the roller as desired, returning to any area with particular tension. Hold for 5 to 30 seconds. Breathe slowly and fully. Switch sides.

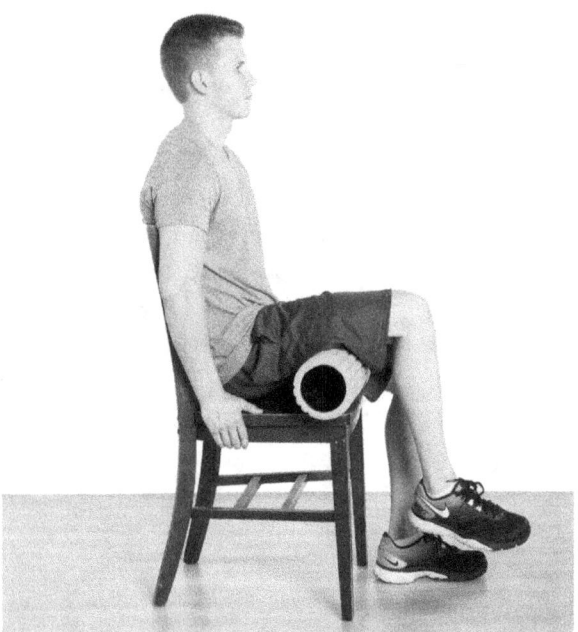

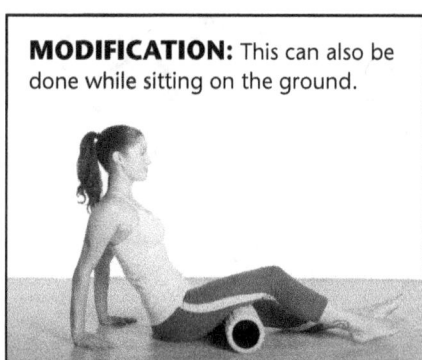

MODIFICATION: This can also be done while sitting on the ground.

This is the starting platform for all lying exercises.

Goal: To acquaint you with the roller

STARTING POSITION: Place a roller on the floor and lie on it from head to tailbone. Place your feet on the floor, with your knees bent and arms out to the side for additional stability.

starting position

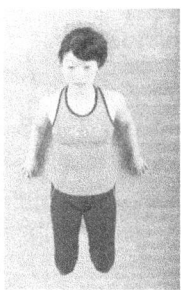

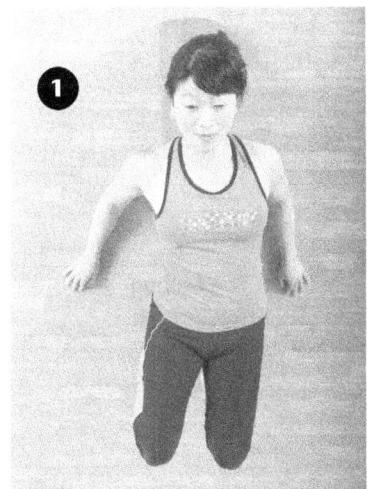

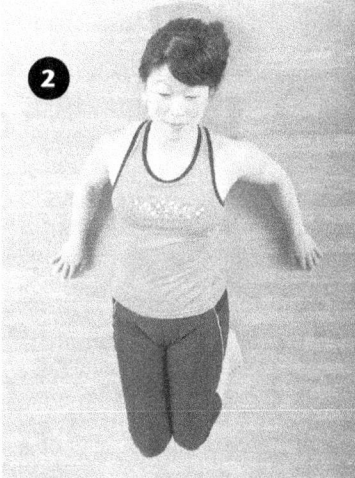

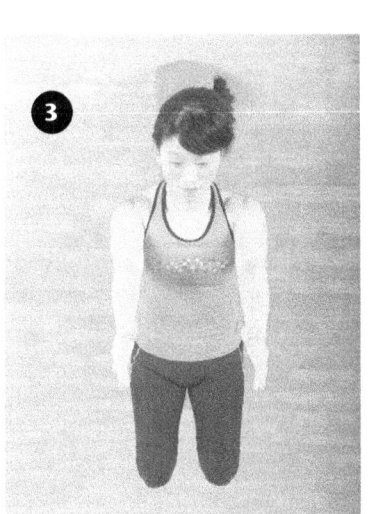

1–2 Once you feel stable, gently roll left and right and recover your balance.

3 Once you feel more stable, try lifting your arms to the ceiling while balancing in the center.

Goal: To strengthen the gluteal region, lower back and legs

CAUTION: Be careful to avoid hamstring cramps.

STARTING POSITION: Place a FLHR flat side down on the floor and lie on it from head to tailbone. Place your feet on the floor, with your knees bent and arms alongside your body.

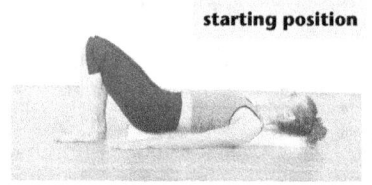

starting position

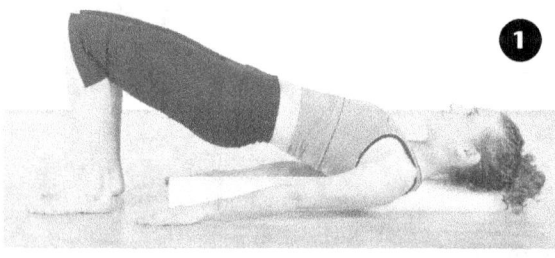

1

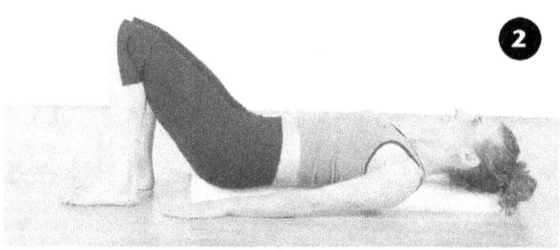

2

1 Slowly lift your rear end off the floor and hold for 5–30 seconds. Avoid going too high and arching your back as this can cause cramping of the hamstring muscles.

2 Lower to starting position.

INTERMEDIATE: Flip the roller over and perform the exercise with the flat side up, or try it on a FLCR.

ADVANCED: Perform this movement with your feet on the roller instead.

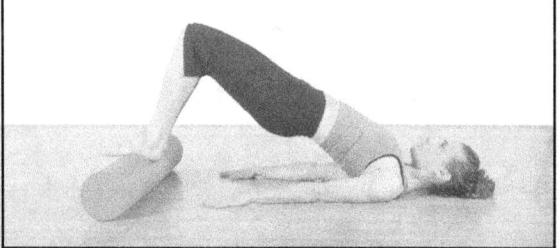

Goal: To strengthen the gluteal region, lower back and legs

CAUTION: Be careful to avoid hamstring cramps.

STARTING POSITION: Place a FLHR flat side down on the floor and lie on it from head to tailbone. Place your feet on the floor with your knees bent and arms alongside your body.

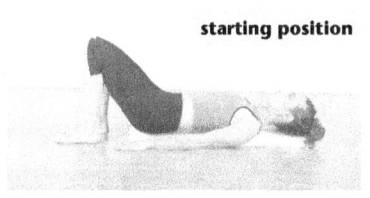

starting position

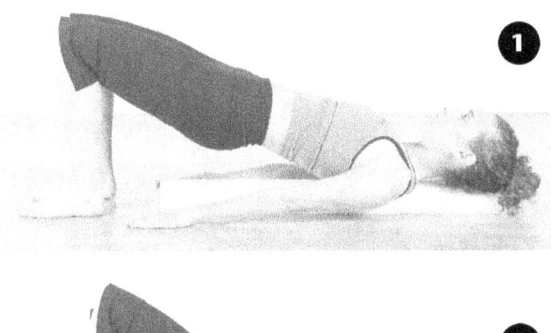

1

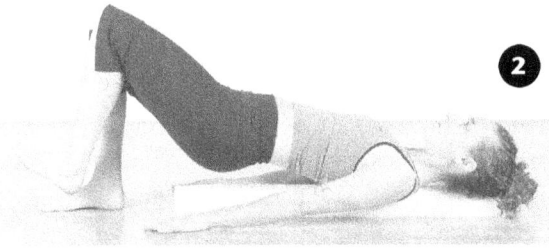

2

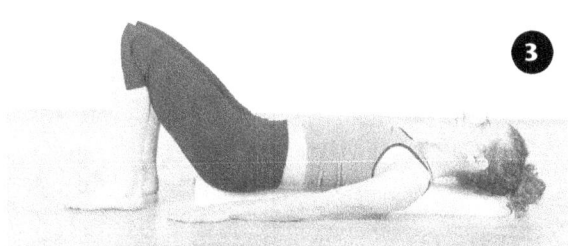

3

1 Slowly lift your rear end off the floor and hold. Avoid going too high and arching your back as this can cause cramping of the hamstring muscles.

2 Once stable, slowly lift your left foot 1–2 inches off the roller and hold.

3 Relax and return to starting position.

Repeat, then switch the foot you lift.

INTERMEDIATE: Flip the roller over and perform the exercise with the flat side up, or try it on a FLCR.

ADVANCED: Try this with your arms across your chest and your feet on a second roller.

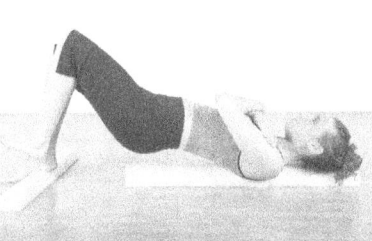

Goal: To improve core stability

STARTING POSITION: Place a FLHR flat side down on the floor and lie on it from head to tailbone. Place your feet on the floor, with your knees bent and arms alongside your body.

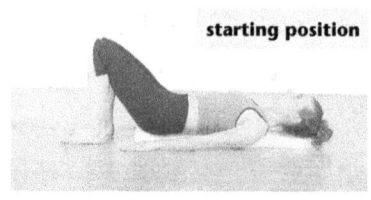

starting position

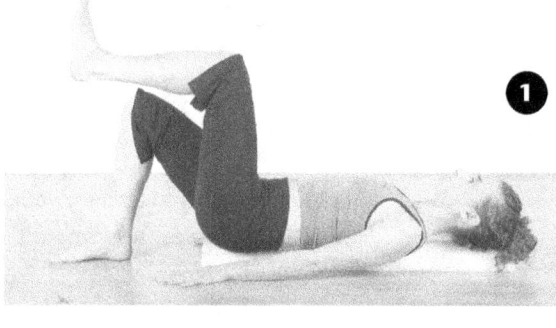

1 Once stable, lift your left leg so that your thigh makes a 90-degree angle with your chest. Hold.

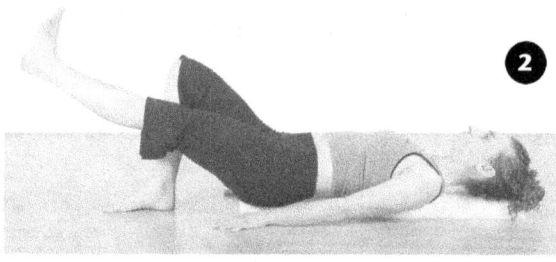

2 Slowly press your leg forward (toward a wall) while maintaining proper position on the roller.

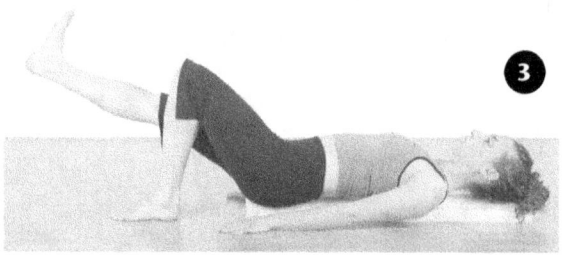

3 Return to starting position then switch sides.

INTERMEDIATE: Flip the roller over and perform the exercise with the flat side up, or try it on a FLCR.

ADVANCED: Start with both legs elevated to 90 degrees.

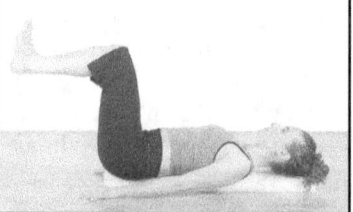

Remember to maintain perfect posture.

Goal: To tone the upper torso and improve core stability

STARTING POSITION: Place a FLHR flat side up under your toes and place your hands on the floor in a push-up position.

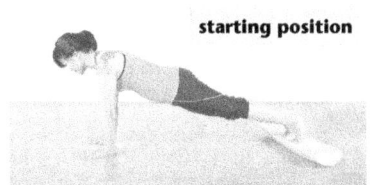
starting position

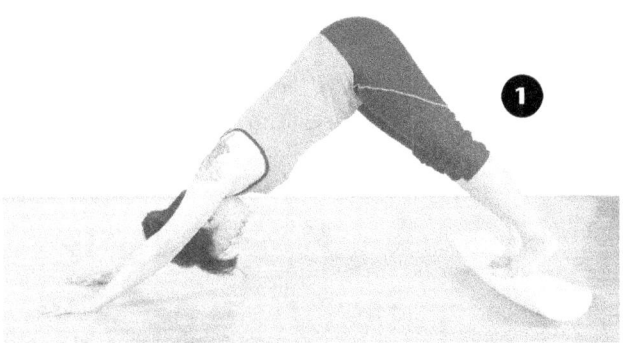
1

1 Once stable, raise your rear end up to a pike position and hold for 5 seconds.

2 Return to starting position and hold for 5 seconds.

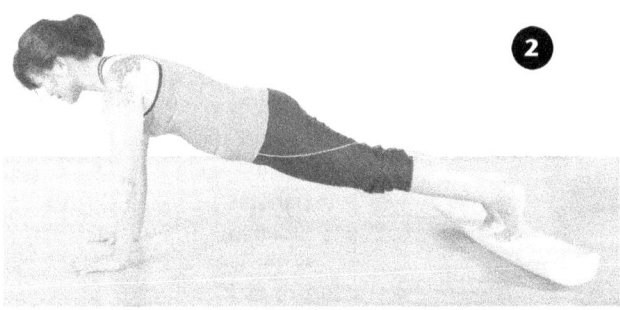
2

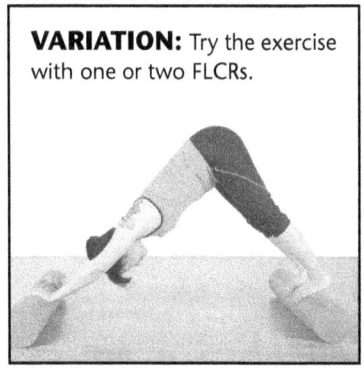
VARIATION: Try the exercise with one or two FLCRs.

This is a very challenging exercise.

Goal: To tone the upper body and torso as well as glutes and adductor muscle in the inner thigh

STARTING POSITION: Position a FLHR flat side down under your chest, then place your hands on the roller and knees on the floor. Once you have your balance, extend your legs behind you and assume a push-up position.

starting position

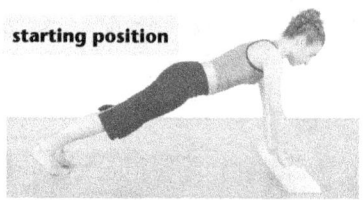

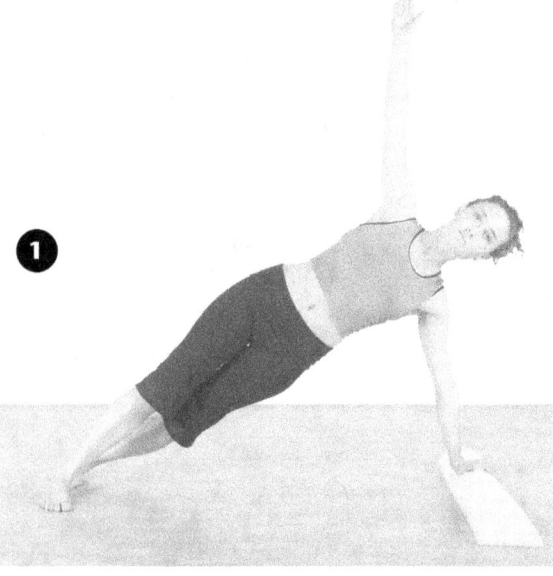

1 Slowly rotate your body to the right, relying only on your left arm to support you. If you can, extend your right arm to the ceiling so that you're in a side plank.

2 Return to starting position.

Now rotate to the other side.

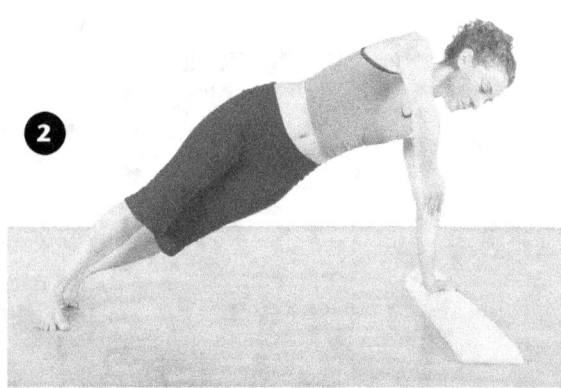

INTERMEDIATE: Each time you return to push-up position, perform 2 push-ups between rotations.

ADVANCED: Flip the roller over and perform the exercise with the flat side up, or try it on a FLCR.

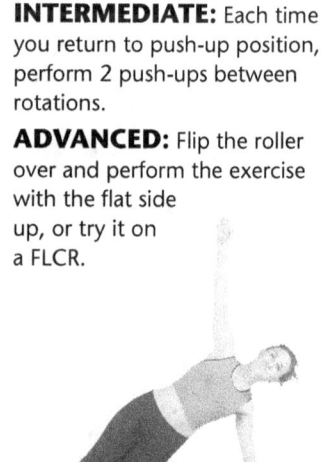

There are three options in this sequence.

Goal: To improve balance and core stability

STARTING POSITION: Place a FLCR under your knees and a second one under your hands.

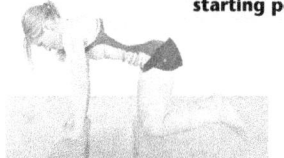

starting position

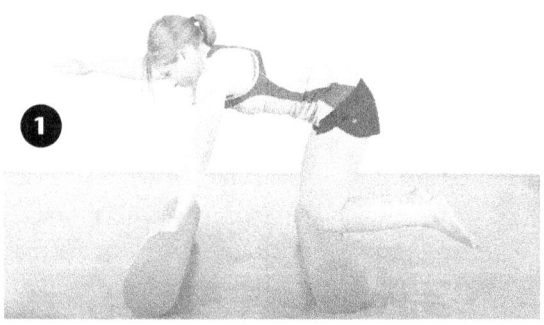

Level 1 (arms only)

1 Once stable and stationary, raise one arm as high as you safely can. Hold.

Switch sides and hold.

Level 2 (legs only)

2 Slowly raise one leg as high as you safely can. Hold.

Switch sides and hold.

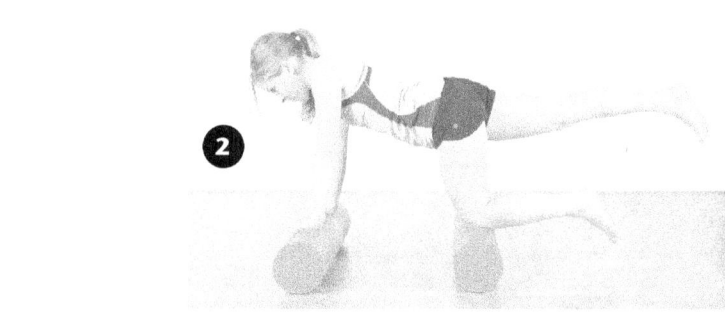

Level 3 (combination)

3 Slowly raise your right arm and left leg. Hold.

Switch sides and hold.

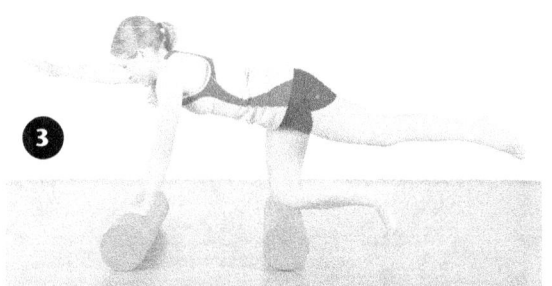

MODIFICATION: If balance is an issue, try this with FLHRs, flat sides down or up.

VARIATION: Place a roller under your right knee and right hand, and another roller under your left hand and left knee. Perform the series.

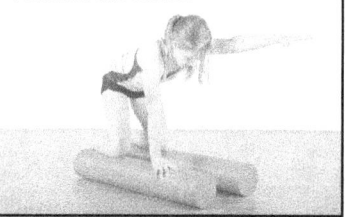

This is considered a basic foundational exercise using the roller.

Goal: To gain familiarity with the roller and improve strength throughout the entire leg, including glutes, quads, hamstrings and calf muscles

STARTING POSITION: Stand with your back to a wall and place a FLCR horizontally between you and the wall, around the level of your lower back.

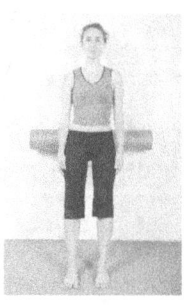

starting position

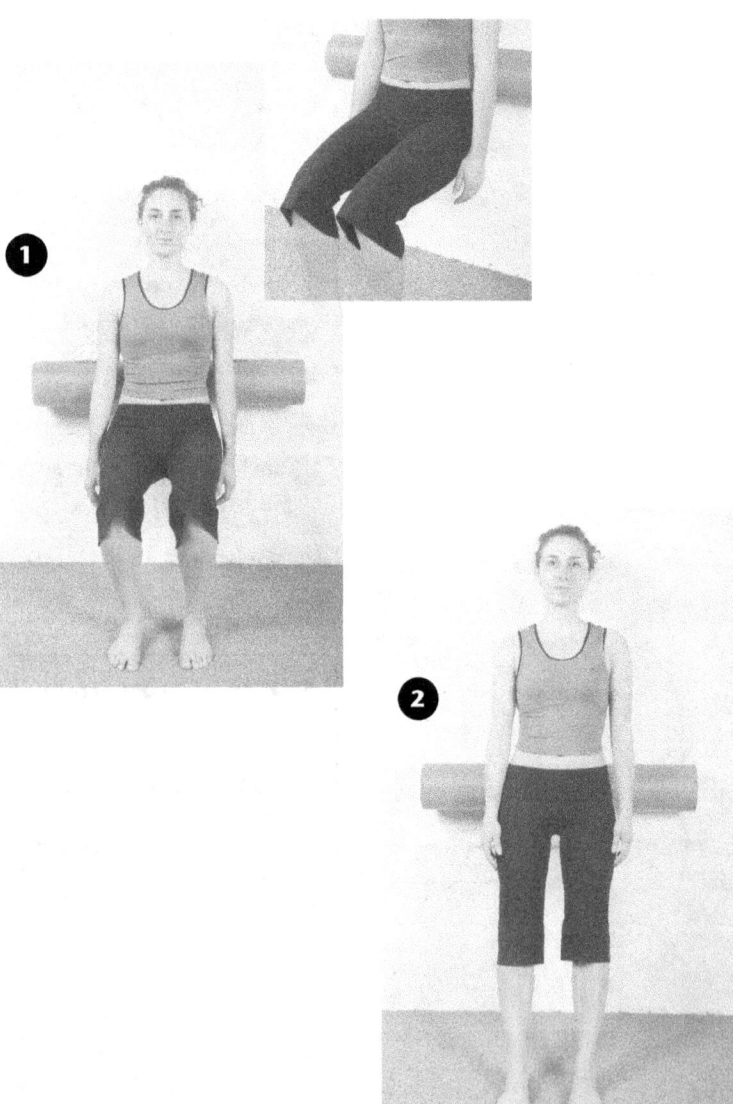

1 Slowly bend your knees to lower yourself halfway to the floor. The roller will roll up your back. Maintain body contact with the roller; the roller must remain in contact with the wall.

2 Return to standing.

This exercise is considered one of the most basic standing moves on a roller.

Goal: To foster core stability and balance and strengthen the calf muscles

CAUTION: If you're unable to maintain proper posture and balance, do not attempt any of the other exercises in the standing series until you can meet this minimum requirement. It's suggested that you return to the seated or kneeling exercises to improve your balance.

STARTING POSITION: Stand with a FLHR flat side down on the floor in front of you.

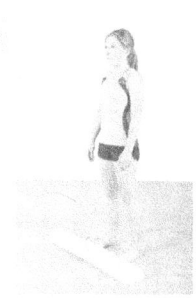

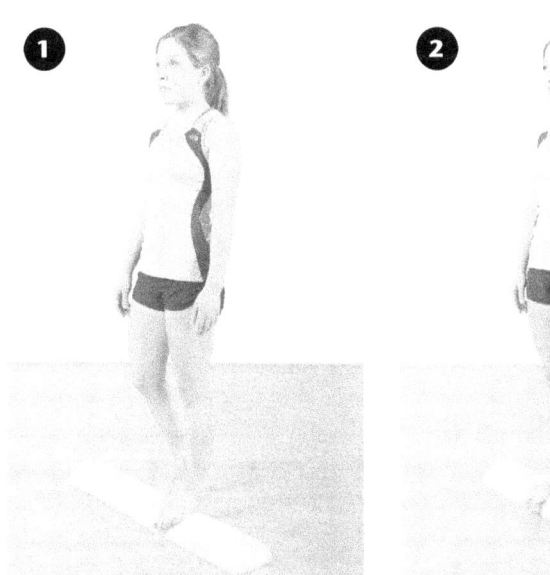

1–2 Step onto the roller with your left foot and then your right. Place your feet shoulder-width apart and maintain proper posture. Hold for 5–30 seconds.

INTERMEDIATE: Flip the roller over and perform the exercise with the flat side up, or try it on a FLCR. This is extremely challenging and should not be performed until you can do the basic exercise for at least 1 minute. BE CAREFUL!

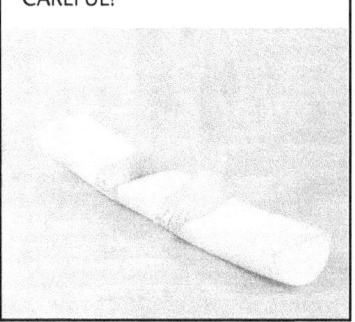

Goal: To improve balance

STARTING POSITION: Stand with a FLHR flat side down on the floor in front of you. Step onto the roller with your left foot and then your right foot; have something to hold on to for additional support if you need it.

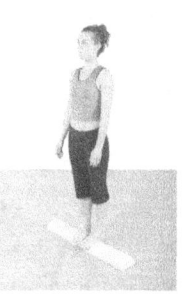

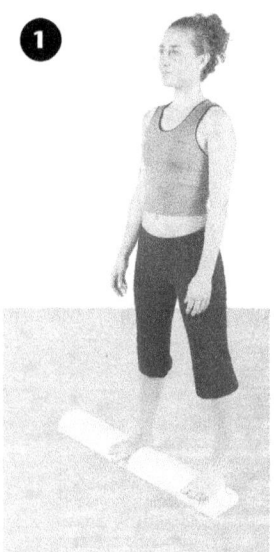

1 Slowly slide your left foot to the left and hold.

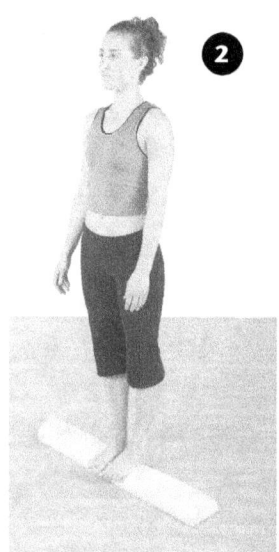

2 Slowly return your left foot to starting position and hold.

3 Slowly slide your right foot to the right and hold.

Continue sliding left and right.

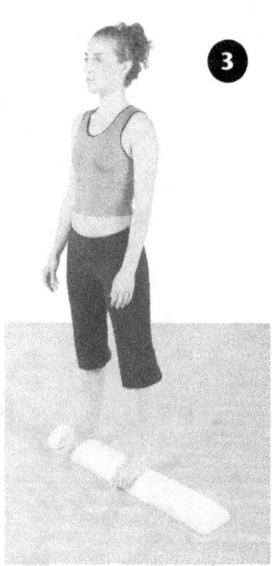

INTERMEDIATE: As you advance, move your foot farther toward the end of the roller.

ADVANCED: Flip the roller over and perform the exercise with the flat side up, or try it on a FLCR. BE CAREFUL!

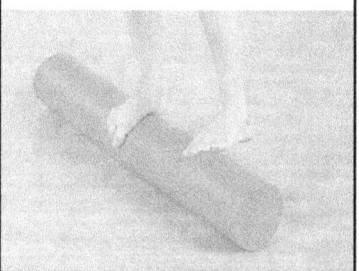

Goal: To improve balance, leg strength and stamina

STARTING POSITION: Place a FLHR flat side down on the floor. Step onto the roller with your left foot and then your right.

starting position

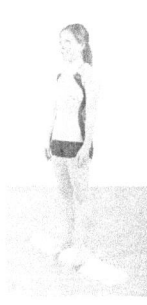

1

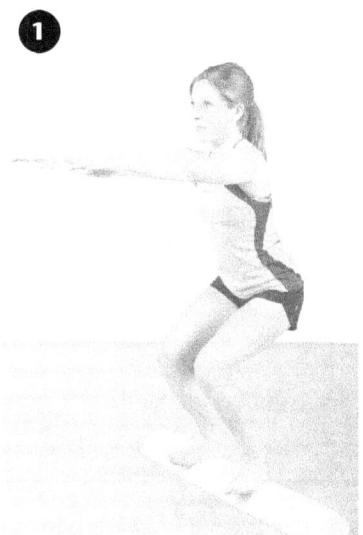

2

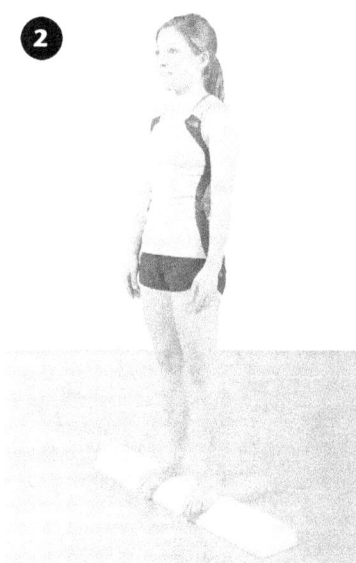

1 Standing in your most stable position and using your hands to counterbalance yourself, slowly perform a small squat.

2 Return to starting position.

INTERMEDIATE: As you improve, try to rely less on your arms for balance by crossing them.

ADVANCED: Flip the roller over and perform the exercise with the flat side up.

SUPER-ADVANCED: Perform the standing mini squat on a FLCR. This is extremely challenging and should not be performed until you can do the basic exercise for at least 1 minute.

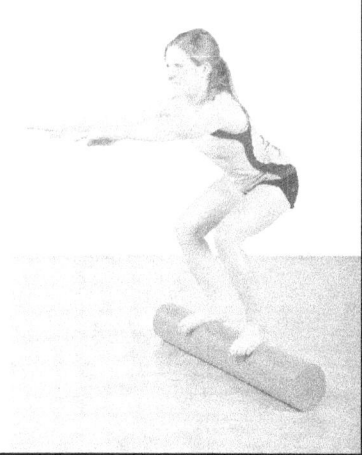

Goal: To foster better balance and core stability and strengthen the entire leg

STARTING POSITION: Stand with a FLHR flat side down on the floor in front of you. Place a large object such as a big balance ball or beach ball in front of it.

starting position

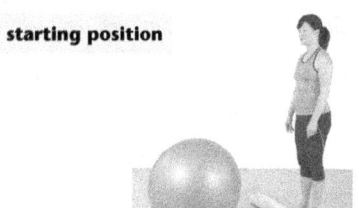

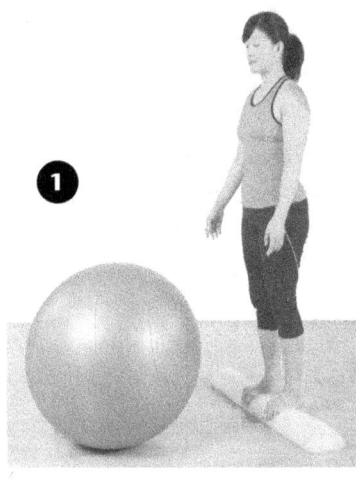

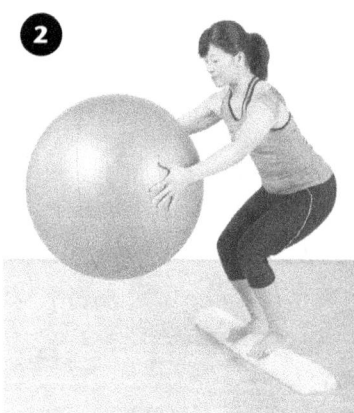

1 Step onto the roller with your left foot and then your right foot.

2 Standing in your most stable position and keeping your back as straight as possible, slowly squat down to pick up the object.

3 Return to standing.

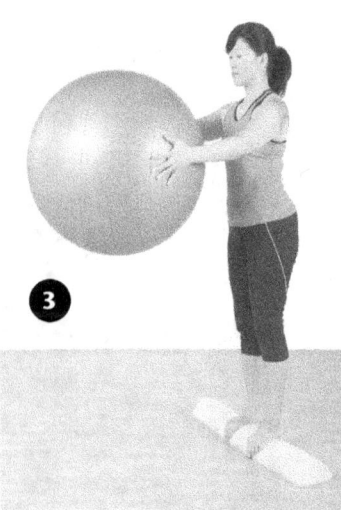

INTERMEDIATE: Flip the roller over and perform the exercise with the flat side up.

ADVANCED: Perform the exercise on a FLCR. BE CAREFUL!

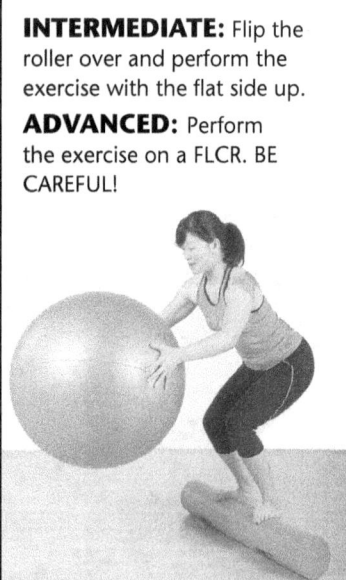

Goal: To improve dynamic balance

STARTING POSITION: Stand with a FLHR flat side down and lengthwise on the floor in front of you. You may need to place a sturdy object/chair next to you for support.

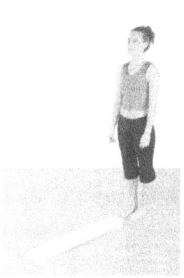

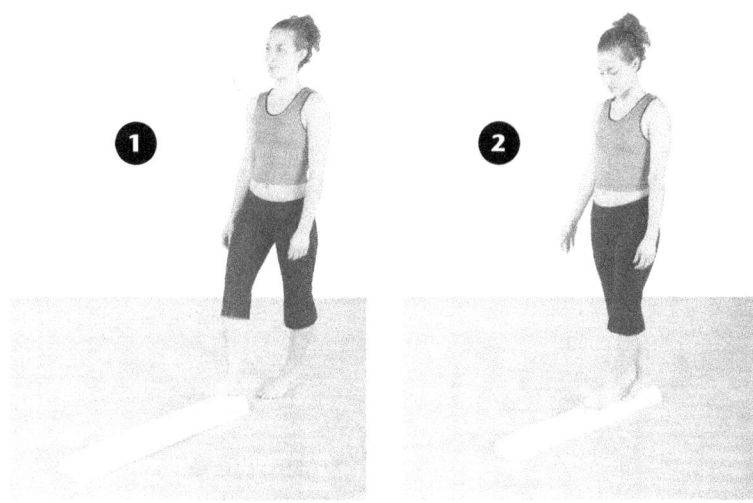

1–2 Attempt to walk the length of the roller, placing one foot in front of the other, heel to toe.

3 Step off, turn around and repeat.

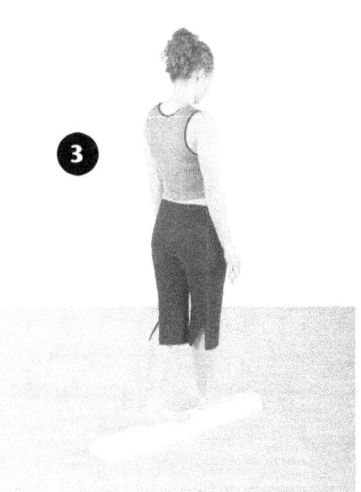

INTERMEDIATE: As you advance, attempt to walk backward or with your eyes closed.

ADVANCED: Flip the roller over and perform the exercise with the flat side up.

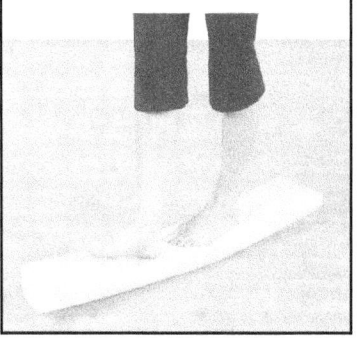

Goal: To improve dynamic balance and ankle flexibility, and to stretch the calf muscles

STARTING POSITION: Stand with a FLHR flat side up on the floor in front of you. You may need to place a sturdy object/chair next to you for support.

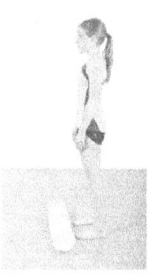

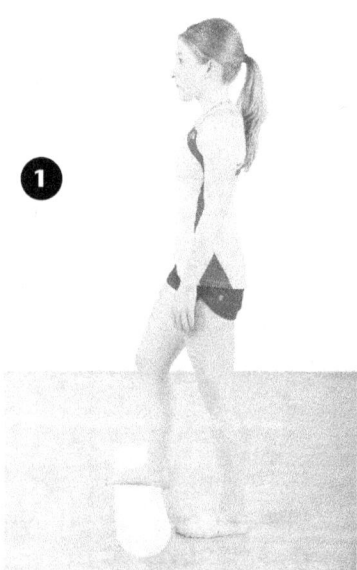

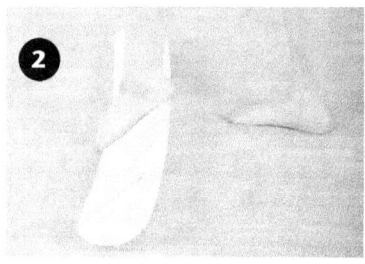

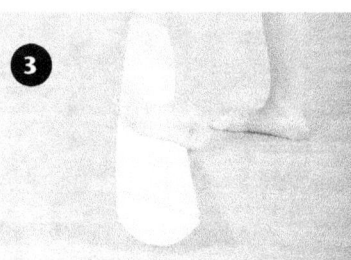

1 Place one foot on the roller.

2–3 Slowly roll your toes forward and then rock your heels back toward the floor.

Switch sides.

VARIATION: For an extra challenge, try this with both feet on the roller.

MODIFICATION: You can perform this exercise while sitting in a chair.

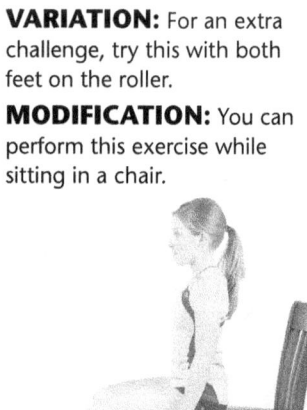

Goal: To strengthen the hip and gluteal region

This is extremely challenging and should not be performed until you can do the previous exercises in this series easily and safely.

STARTING POSITION: Place a FLHR flat side down between your feet so that you're straddling the roller. You may need to place a sturdy object/chair next to you for support.

starting position

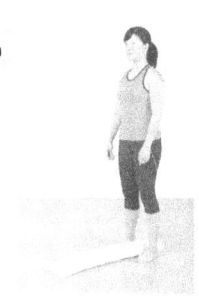

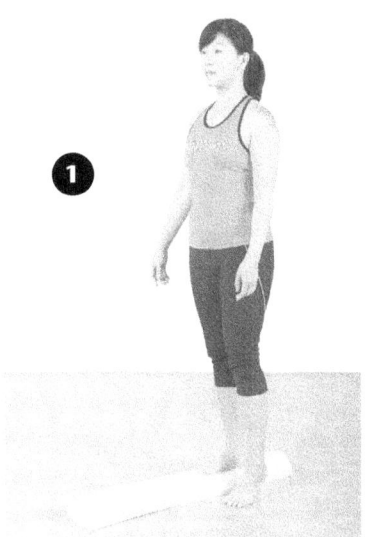

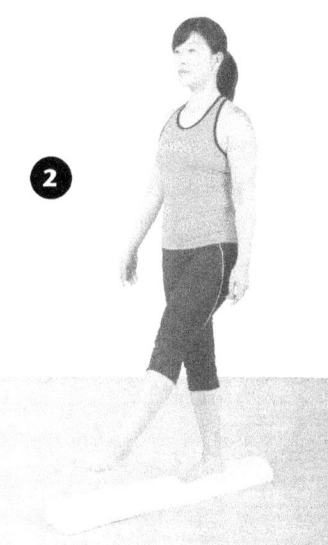

1 Place your right foot on the roller while allowing your left foot to provide as much stability as required.

2 While maintaining your balance, raise your left foot and stand only on your right foot for at least 15 seconds.

Switch sides.

VARIATION: For an extra challenge, try this with the flat side up.

MODIFICATION: Use a chair for support if you have balance issues.

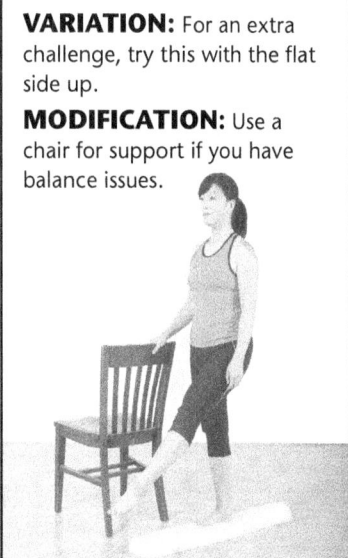

Goal: To learn to distribute your weight evenly

STARTING POSITION: Stand with two FLHRs side by side (shoulder-width apart) on the floor, flat sides down. You may need to place a sturdy object/chair next to you for support.

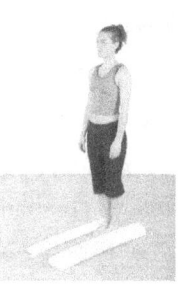

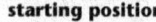

1 Place one foot on one roller and the other foot on the other roller, as if skiing. Maintain balance and proper posture and hold.

INTERMEDIATE: As you advance, slowly shift your weight from one side to the other and hold for 30–60 seconds.

You can also try it with your eyes closed.

ADVANCED: Flip the rollers over and perform the exercise with the flat sides up.

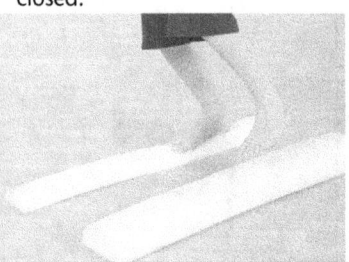

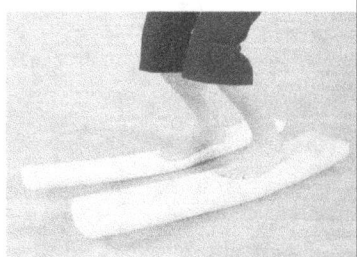

Goal: To learn to distribute your weight evenly while performing strength and conditioning exercises

STARTING POSITION: Stand with two FLHRs side by side (shoulder-width apart) on the floor, flat sides down. You may need to place a sturdy object/chair next to you for support. Place one foot on one roller

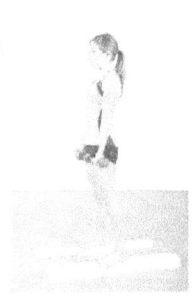

starting position

and the other foot on the other roller, as if skiing.

1 Maintain balance and proper posture as you perform arm curls (with or without light handweights).

2 Perform lateral raises (with or without light handweights).

3 Perform frontal raises (with or without light handweights).

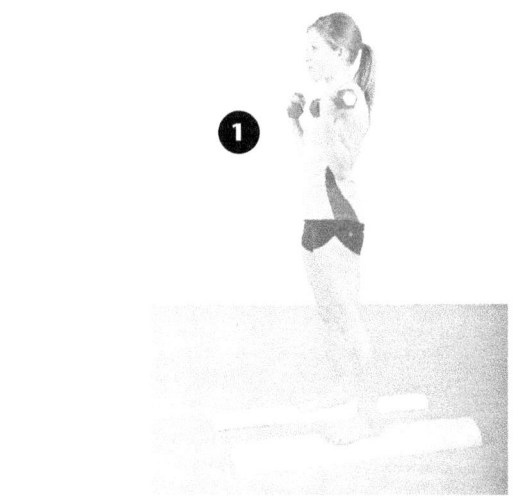

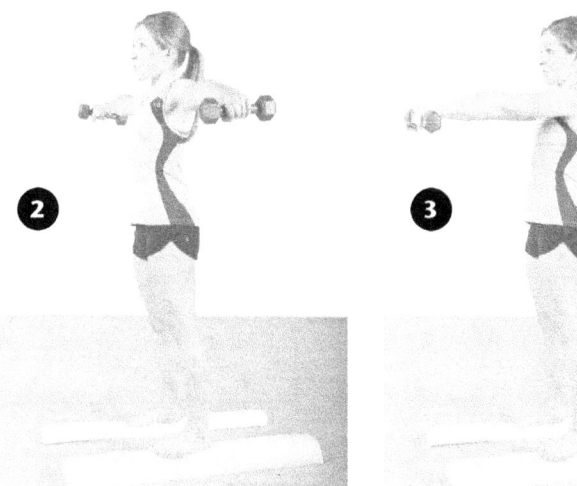

> **VARIATION:** Flip the rollers over and perform the motions with the flat sides up.

Goal: To improve circulation and release tight gluteal muscles

STARTING POSITION: Sit on a FLCR that's either placed horizontally on the floor or a chair. Shift your weight so that you're on one butt cheek.

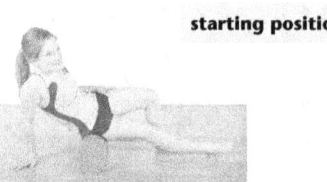

starting position

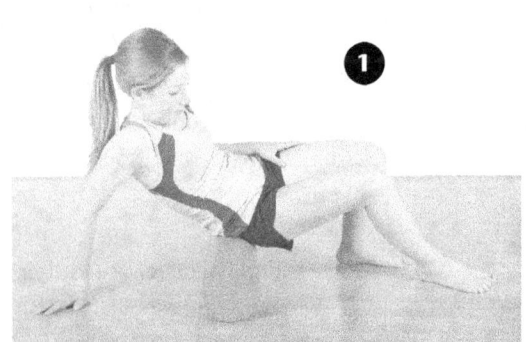

1

1–2 Slowly roll your rear end forward then backward, stopping at any point along the way that requires a little more attention. You can also slowly lean to the left and hold, and then shift your weight to the right.

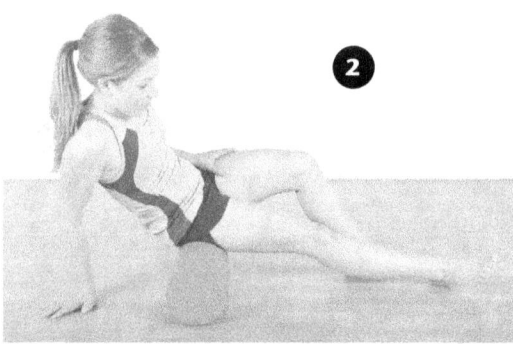

2

Goal: To relieve tight thigh muscles

STARTING POSITION: Lie face down and place a FLCR under your thighs. Place your hands on the floor for support.

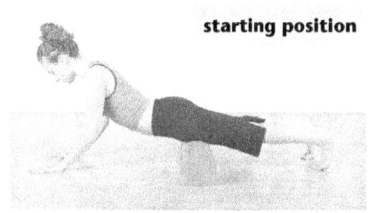

starting position

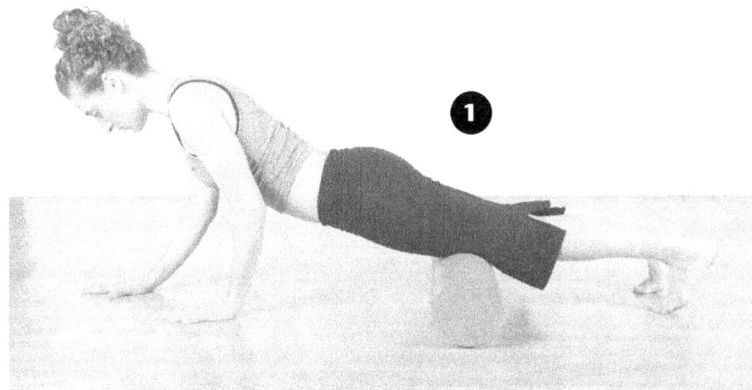

1 Slowly roll the roller down toward the knee area. Do not roll on or over the knees.

2 Slowly roll the roller back up toward your hips, stopping at spots along the way that require more attention.

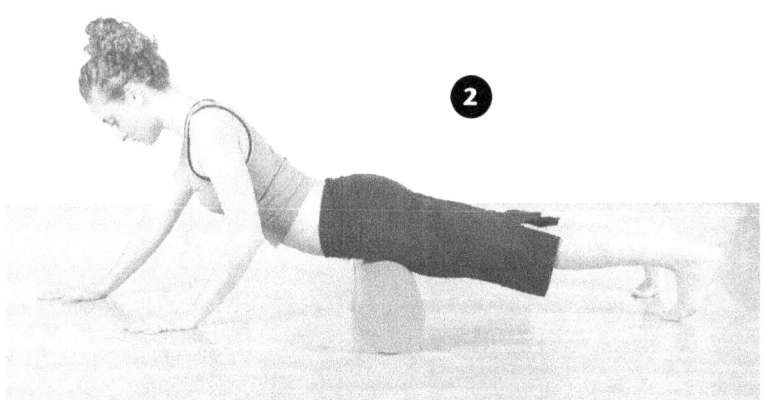

STARTING POSITION: While kneeling, place the knobbed roller on your thighs, close to your hip crease.

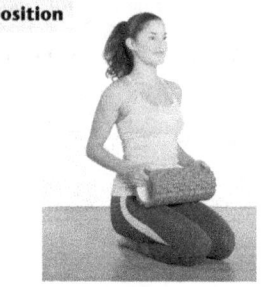

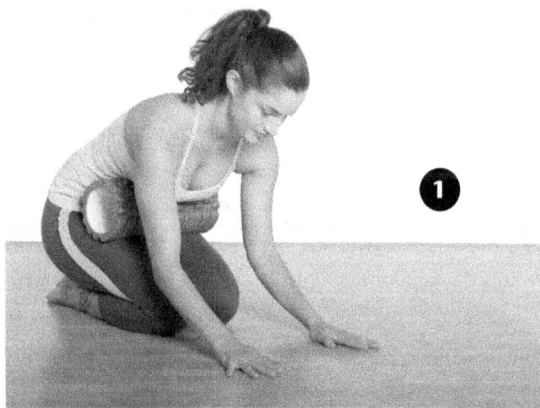

1–2 Slowly and gradually fold over the roller, reaching forward with your arms. Breathe slowly and fully, letting your muscles relax.

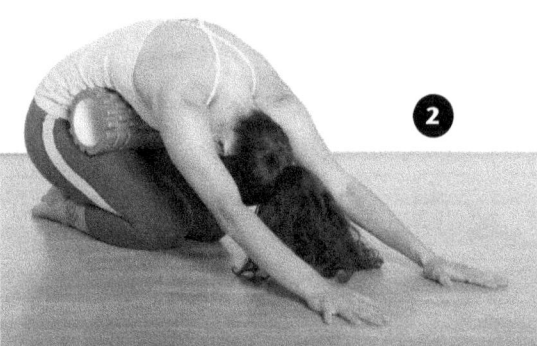

Goal: To massage the IT band/upper-outer thigh

STARTING POSITION: Lie on one side and place a FLCR under your bottom leg. Use your hands and other foot for support.

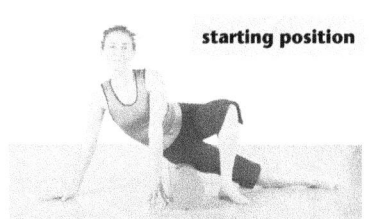
starting position

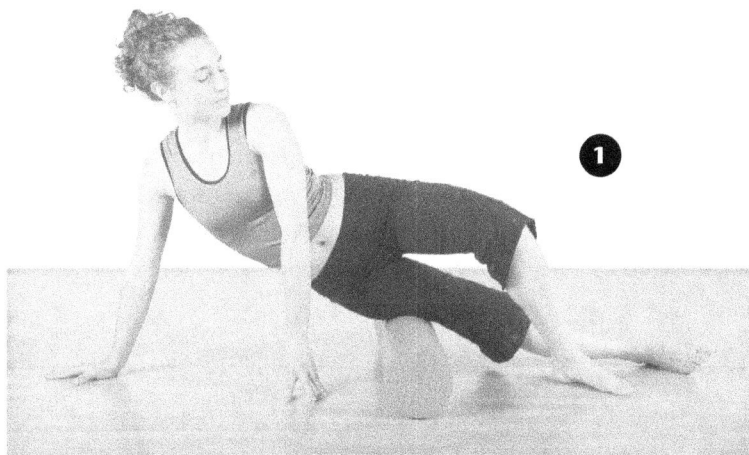

1 Starting just below the hip bone, slowly roll the roller toward, but stop just above, the knee.

2 Slowly roll the roller back up toward the hip, stopping at spots along the way that require more attention.

Switch sides.

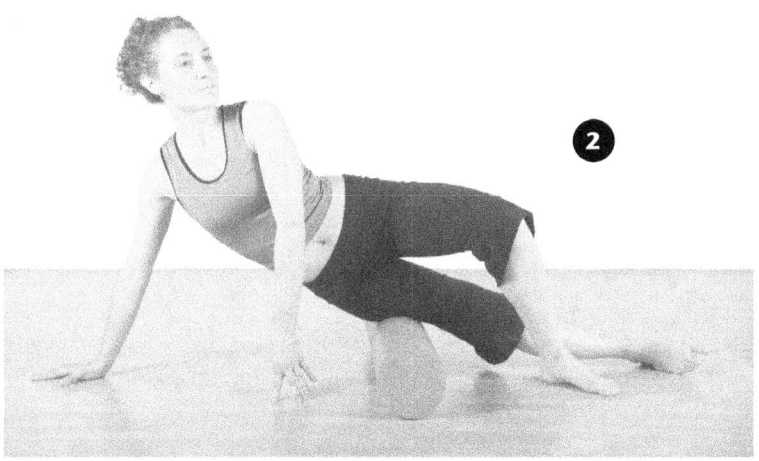

VARIATION: You can also pause at a tight spot and rock from side to side.

Goal: To massage the inner thigh muscles

STARTING POSITION: Lie on one side and place a FLCR between your thighs. You can keep your leg straight or slightly bent.

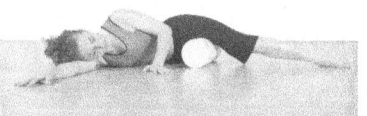

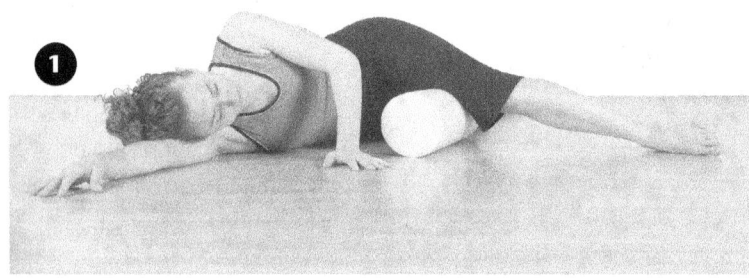

1 Slowly and gently roll your top leg up and down the roller. Along the way, stop and apply gentle pressure wherever additional attention is needed.

Switch sides.

VARIATION: While lying on your side, you can also place the roller between your thighs and let gravity do the work.

This can be performed on one or both calves at the same time.

STARTING POSITION: Sit with your legs extended, propping yourself up on your elbows and/or hands. Place the knobbed roller at the top of your calf muscle near the knee.

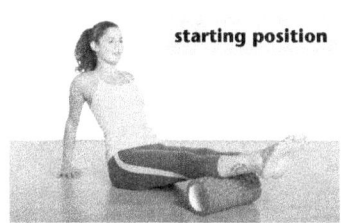

starting position

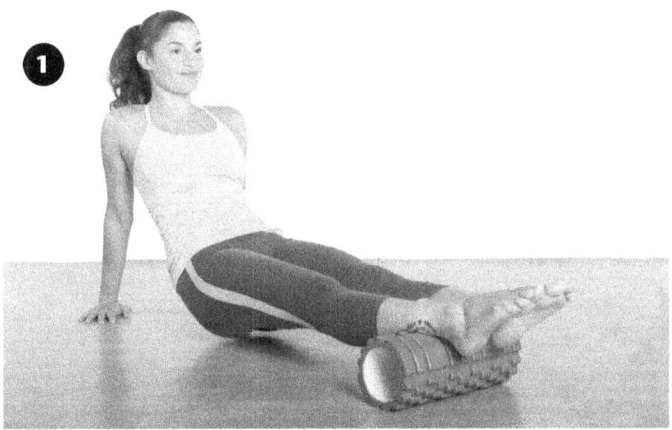

1 Using your arms to move your legs, slowly roll the roller up and down the backs of your calves. Hold at tender locations as needed.

Switch sides.

VARIATION: You can also turn your foot inward and outward to get the inside and outside of the calf.

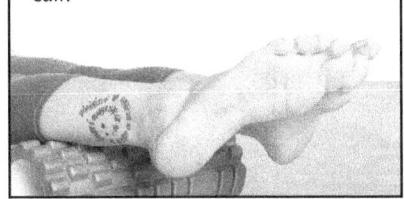

MODIFICATION: This can also be done while lying faceup.

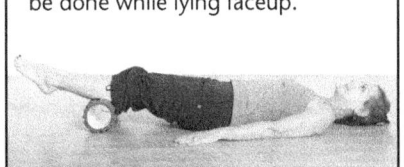

Goal: To massage tight hamstrings

STARTING POSITION: Sit on the floor with one knee bent and the other leg straight. Place a FLCR horizontally beneath the hamstring of your straight leg.

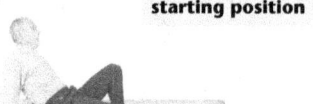

starting position

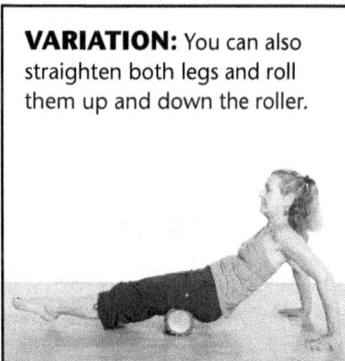

1 Slowly roll the leg up and down the roller. Along the way, stop wherever additional attention is needed and apply just enough pressure to release tension.

Switch sides.

VARIATION: You can also straighten both legs and roll them up and down the roller.

Goal: To massage the arches of your feet and prevent or relieve plantar fasciitis

STARTING POSITION: Sit in a chair and place both feet in the middle of a FLCR.

starting position

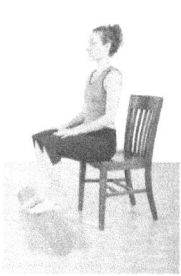

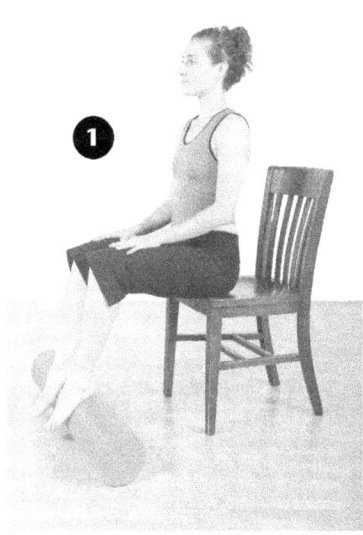

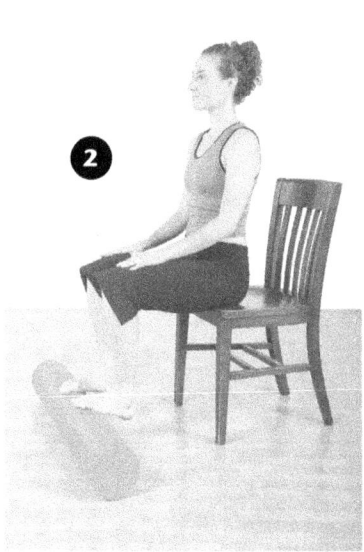

1–2 Slowly roll your feet forward and then backward to massage the arches and bottoms of your feet. Along the way, stop and apply additional pressure where needed.

FOAM ROLLER LOG

Day:_____ **Date:**_____

MUSCLES WORKED ON (Illustrate)	EXERCISE
(A)	
(B)	
(C)	
(D)	
(E)	
(F)	
(G)	
(H)	

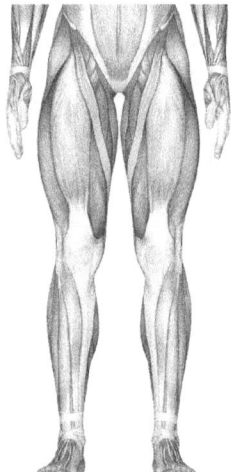 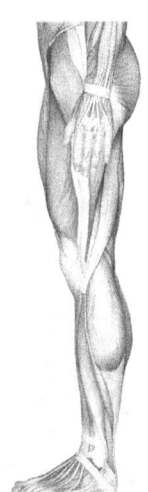 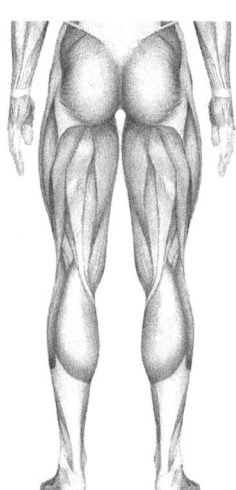

NOTES:

HOW ARE YOUR LEGS FEELING TODAY?

Poor ← 1   2   3   4   5   6   7   8   9   10 → Great

FOAM ROLLER LOG

Day:_____ **Date:**_____

MUSCLES WORKED ON (Illustrate)	EXERCISE
(A)	
(B)	
(C)	
(D)	
(E)	
(F)	
(G)	
(H)	

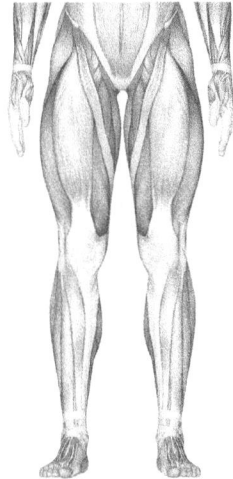 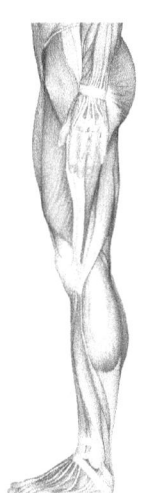 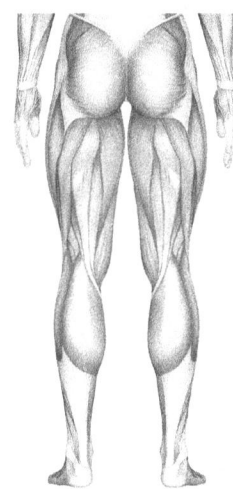

NOTES:

HOW ARE YOUR LEGS FEELING TODAY?

Poor ← 1   2   3   4   5   6   7   8   9   10 → Great

FOAM ROLLER LOG

Day:_____ **Date:**_____

MUSCLES WORKED ON (Illustrate)	EXERCISE
(A)	
(B)	
(C)	
(D)	
(E)	
(F)	
(G)	
(H)	

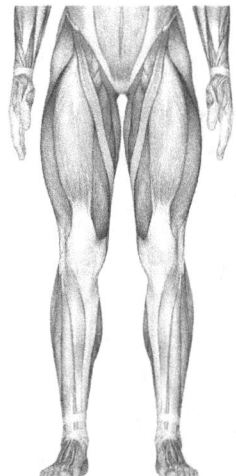 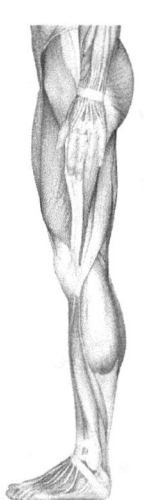 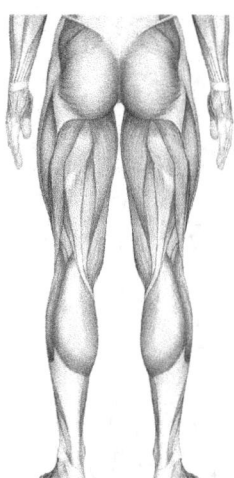

NOTES:

HOW ARE YOUR LEGS FEELING TODAY?

Poor ← 1   2   3   4   5   6   7   8   9   10 → Great

FOAM ROLLER LOG

Day:_____ **Date:**_____

MUSCLES WORKED ON (Illustrate)	EXERCISE
(A)	
(B)	
(C)	
(D)	
(E)	
(F)	
(G)	
(H)	

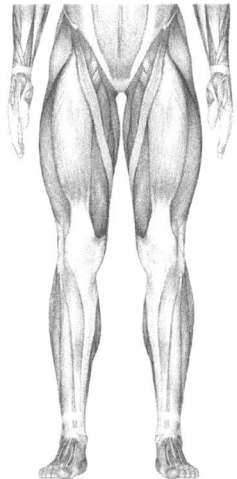 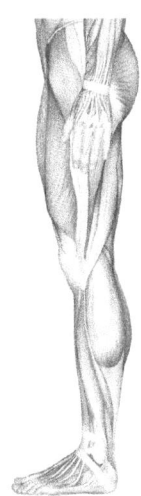 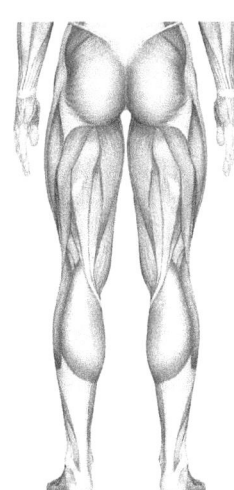

NOTES:

HOW ARE YOUR LEGS FEELING TODAY?

Poor ← 1   2   3   4   5   6   7   8   9   10 → Great

FOAM ROLLER LOG

Day:_____ **Date:**_____

MUSCLES WORKED ON (Illustrate)	EXERCISE
(A)	
(B)	
(C)	
(D)	
(E)	
(F)	
(G)	
(H)	

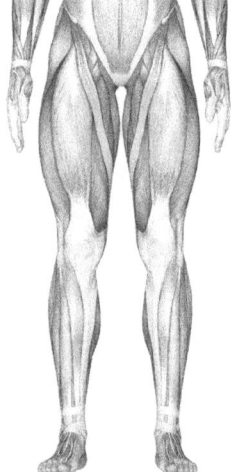 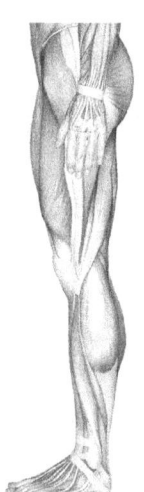 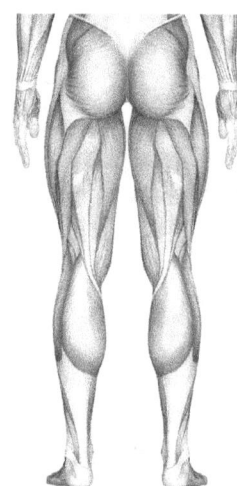

NOTES:

HOW ARE YOUR LEGS FEELING TODAY?

Poor ← 1   2   3   4   5   6   7   8   9   10 → Great

FOAM ROLLER LOG

Day:_____ **Date:**_____

MUSCLES WORKED ON (Illustrate)	EXERCISE
(A)	
(B)	
(C)	
(D)	
(E)	
(F)	
(G)	
(H)	

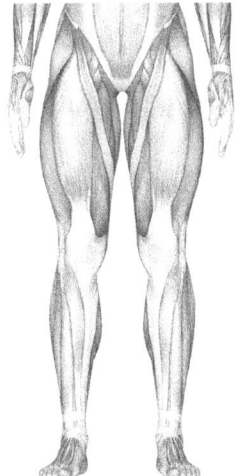 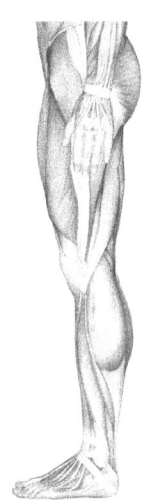 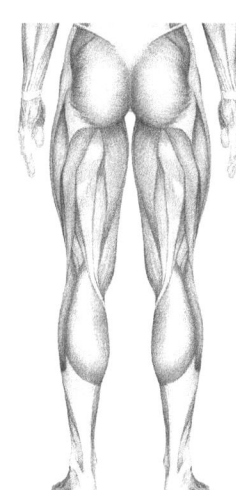

NOTES:

HOW ARE YOUR LEGS FEELING TODAY?

Poor ← 1   2   3   4   5   6   7   8   9   10 → Great

FOAM ROLLER LOG

Day:_____ **Date:**_____

MUSCLES WORKED ON (Illustrate)	EXERCISE
(A)	
(B)	
(C)	
(D)	
(E)	
(F)	
(G)	
(H)	

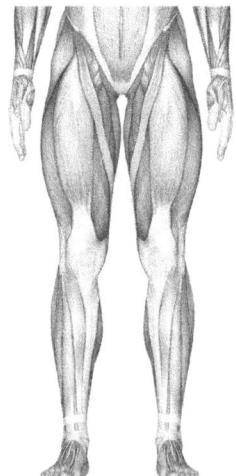 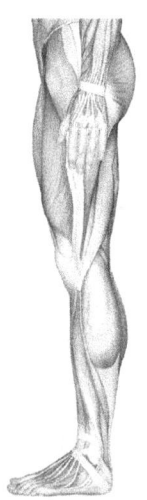 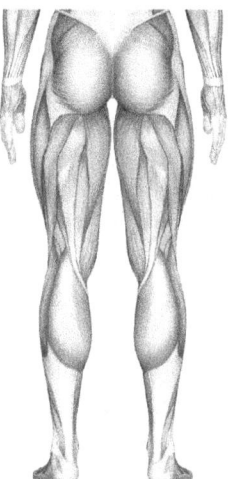

NOTES:

HOW ARE YOUR LEGS FEELING TODAY?

Poor ← 1   2   3   4   5   6   7   8   9   10 → Great

FOAM ROLLER LOG

Day:_____ **Date:**_____

MUSCLES WORKED ON (Illustrate)	EXERCISE
(A)	
(B)	
(C)	
(D)	
(E)	
(F)	
(G)	
(H)	

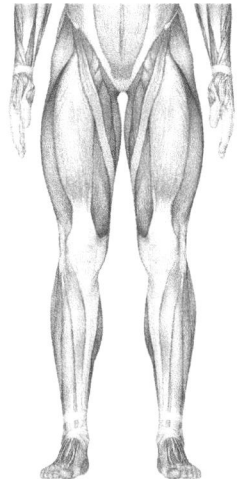 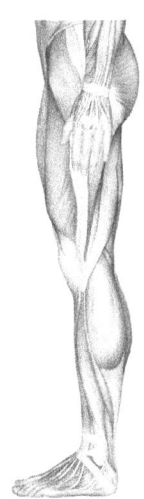 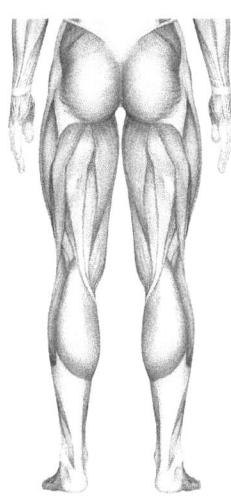

NOTES:

HOW ARE YOUR LEGS FEELING TODAY?

Poor ← 1   2   3   4   5   6   7   8   9   10 → Great

FOAM ROLLER LOG

Day:_____ **Date:**_____

MUSCLES WORKED ON (Illustrate)	EXERCISE
(A)	
(B)	
(C)	
(D)	
(E)	
(F)	
(G)	
(H)	

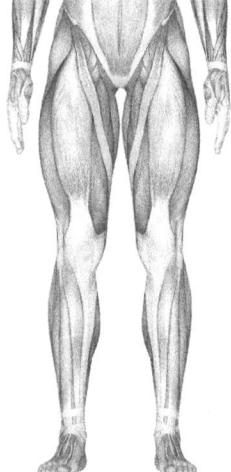
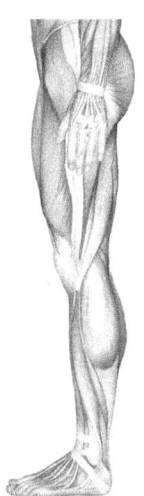
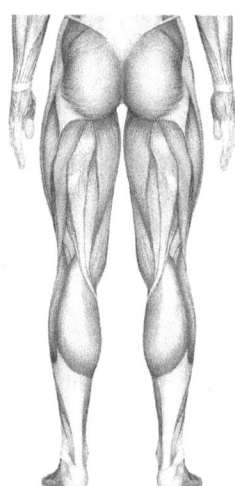

NOTES:

HOW ARE YOUR LEGS FEELING TODAY?

Poor ⟵ 1   2   3   4   5   6   7   8   9   10 ⟶ Great

FOAM ROLLER LOG

Day:_____ **Date:**_____

MUSCLES WORKED ON (Illustrate)	EXERCISE
(A)	
(B)	
(C)	
(D)	
(E)	
(F)	
(G)	
(H)	

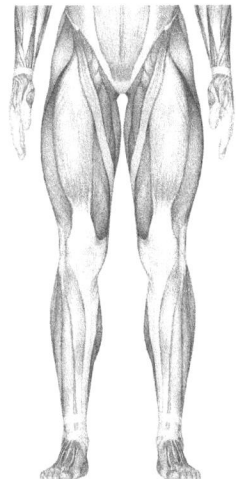 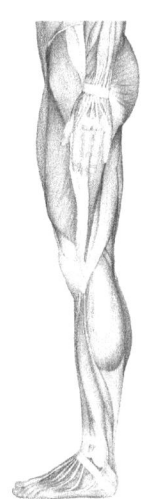 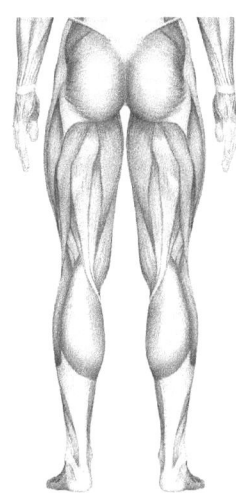

NOTES:

HOW ARE YOUR LEGS FEELING TODAY?

Poor ← 1   2   3   4   5   6   7   8   9   10 → Great

about the author

DR. KARL KNOPF, author of *Healthy Hips Handbook*, *Healthy Shoulder Handbook*, *Stretching for 50+*, *Foam Roller Workbook*, *Trigger Point Therapy with the Foam Roller* and *Injury Rehab with Resistance Bands*, has been involved with the health and fitness of the disabled and older adults for more than 40 years. During this time he has worked in almost every aspect of the industry, from personal training and therapy to consultation.

While at Foothill College, Karl was the coordinator of the Adaptive Fitness Technician Program and Life Long Learning Institute. He taught disabled students and undergraduates about corrective exercise. In addition to teaching, Karl developed the "Fitness Educators of Older Adults Association" to guide trainers of older adults. Currently Karl is a director at the International Sports Science Association.

In his spare time he has spoken at conferences, authored many articles, and written numerous books on topics ranging from water workouts to fitness therapy. He was a frequent guest and currently is board member to PBS's *Sit and Be Fit* show as well as a regular advisor on both radio and print media on issues pertaining to senior fitness and the disabled.

www.ingramcontent.com/pod-product-compliance
Lightning Source LLC
Chambersburg PA
CBHW080438290526
45791CB00008BA/2541